Dr. Deanna's *Healing Handbook*

Natural Aging and Disease Prevention through a Whole Foods
Diet, Hormone Balance, Total Body Detox and Exercise

Deanna Osborn, DO

with Dr. Linda Jeffrey

Cover Photos: © 2014 Nina & Wes Photography
Illustrations: © 2014 Spencer McCloy
Makeup: Maggie Fink

For more information: www.deannaosborn.com

Printed in the United States of America
ISBN: 978-0-9849560-2-9

A Word of Caution to the Reader

The information presented in this book is based on the training and professional
experience of the authors. The treatments recommended in this book should not
be undertaken without first consulting a physician. Proper laboratory and clinical
monitoring is essential to achieving the goals of finding safe and natural treatments.
This book was written for informational and educational purposes only. It is not
intended to be used as medical advice.

Acknowledgements:

Acknowledgements begin with the pioneers John Lee M.D. and David Zava Ph. D. for their research and discoveries in the area of bio-identical hormone balancing, which began my own health restoration, inspired my writing career, and my move toward practicing functional medicine and nutritional healing. Special thanks goes to Eunice Van Winkle Ray for her constant encouragement and her guidance into publishing this work as a vital tool for patient education. New in this expanded edition is the addition of Dr. Linda Jeffrey with her prodigious research capability to expand the reach and depth of the message here. Thank you to the book's other contributors: Dr. Barbara Beaty, Maureen McDonnell, Chef Pam Leveritt, Tara Johnson, Lanty O'Conner and then to D'Etta Thomas, Anna Joy Jeffrey and Gary Kehoe whose testimonials illustrate the real possibility of regaining one's health and wellbeing naturally.

Dedication:

This ongoing work is dedicated to my three children, Christopher, Lauren and Rachel. God blessed each of you with amazing capacities and the courage to respectfully question and verify what is presented to you as fact rather than blindly following along. Today it is not always healthy or right just to accept what we are taught. It is my prayer that all three of you bravely continue to develop the ability to question the status quo, to view things from your own studied and well informed perspective and then move out confidently beyond the boundaries of the box. One of my greatest blessings has been to pass the gracious Wisdom of God onto each of you. Love, Mom

Table of Contents

Prologue
What Does Healthy Feel Like?

Odd question you say, but ask yourself: Do you have the same vigor and energy you had just a few years ago? Do you look at your aging body and declining energy as simply the evidence of the passage of years? Please know, most people should have a much higher level of health and wellbeing, which is achievable by following a few simple guidelines. This handbook is designed to provide an overview of what it feels like to be healthy and how to live a more vital life.

My aim is to help your body operate at peak levels, age naturally and avoid disease. My understanding of health and wellbeing has changed since I began to practice medicine. Over the past ten years, I have learned more about "alternative" health and disease prevention than I did in the traditional study of medicine at school. It is my hope that this handbook will equip others to know how to make well-informed decisions about their life and health maintenance, keeping them from poor operational function and ultimately disease.

In *Ultraprevention*, Dr. Mark Hyman lays out the simple myths about modern medicine: (1) Your doctor knows best, (2) If you have a diagnosis, you know what is wrong with you, (3) Drugs cure disease, (4) Your genes determine your fate, (5) Getting older means aging, (6) Fat is a four letter word, (7) You can get all the vitamins you need from food. I agree with Dr. Hyman:

- You are the one who often knows more than a doctor about your health position and should implement a consistent daily maintenance diet and lifestyle program.

- If you are being treated for a disease condition, the situation causing your problem may not be adequately or thoroughly addressed by the diagnosis or the prescribed treatment or meds. Better nutritional support works wonders – often better than meds - as you will see later in the handbook. If you are toxic, malnourished or vitamin and mineral deficient and/or hormone imbalanced, these conditions can be causal or mask symptoms that would allow your health practitioner to identify the disease process.

1

- Again, drugs too often treat symptoms and not causal factors.
- We are all born with genetic triggers that can predispose us to serious illness, but those triggers are most often "pulled" by environmental factors and our own nutrition and lifestyle habits.
- Aging is largely misunderstood even by doctors: You were designed to go the distance and to be vital and disease-free from womb to tomb.
- Fats are misunderstood. There are good and bad fats. You need the good ones, like Omega 3s, to heal and feed your body. We eliminate good fats from our diets at great peril to our health and wellbeing.

Food should be a restorative and healing fuel for the body, not for comfort, relief, or social entertainment in a high-pressure society. You are going to see from what follows here that this can be the saddest and most difficult truth to accept: Food will either take you up or down. Today the food system is compromised. The nutrition required by all of us for health and wellbeing is becoming harder and harder to access commercially. Knowing your farmers, meat producers, and other food providers is becoming critical to maintaining health and avoiding chronic diseases of the industrialized world.

My advice to you, as a doctor, is to read this short handbook from cover to cover. Use the "Table of Contents," as needed, to become informed and to refresh your understanding, as health is primarily a matter of good practices and habits. If you get off track, get right back on track – tomorrow never comes. Trust that my team and I have read the latest books and surveyed the literature and most important recent research on health and wellbeing. When it is all distilled and analyzed, recurring themes leading to real health are confirmed repeatedly. If you will balance your hormones, reduce your body's toxic load, correct your extensive and pervasive nutritional deficiencies by eating a whole food plant based diet and limiting sugars and simple carbs, inflammation will decrease, cardiac function will improve, metabolic function will stabilize, immunity will be stronger, neurological function will be sharper, and the body will restore itself to your best possible health position.

The truths and challenges contained herein are fundamental and provide a clear statement of where we are today in accessing the necessary elements of good health for both mind and body. Let's get started. You are the one in charge of your health position. Remember you are fearfully and wonderfully made – designed to go the distance – and finally thank you. I am humbled at the thought I might influence your good health through these pages. Here's to your better life!

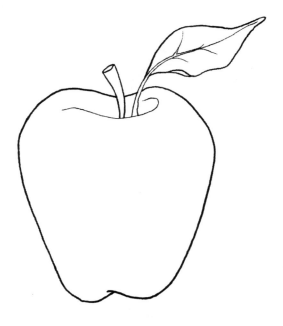

Chapter 1
How Food Has Changed

The Problem is Recent

I often hear the argument, "Well, Grandma never took supplements and she lived to be 95." This is based on the false hypothesis that your health depends entirely on your genetic make-up. So, if Grandma was healthy, you will be too. Yes, your genes matter, but the trigger points for chronic illness such as diabetes and heart disease are clearly directed by what you are feeding your body. And it is a fact that the food your Grandma fed her body is no longer widely available to you. Food has changed nutritionally, genetically, and chemically.

Food Is Less Nutritious

Scientific American published an article in 2011 titled "Dirt Poor" which explains how soil depletion has made our food less nutritious. They report,

> *Modern intensive agricultural methods have stripped increasing amounts of nutrients from the soil in which the food we eat grows. Sadly, each successive generation of fast-growing, pest-resistant carrot is truly less good for you than the one before.*

Scientific American cites a study published in the Journal of the American College of Nutrition that studied U.S. Department of Agriculture nutritional data from 1950 and 1999 for 43 different vegetables and fruits, identifying declines in the amount of protein, calcium, phosphorus, iron, riboflavin, and vitamin C. The study concludes, "Efforts to breed new varieties of crops that provide greater yield, pest resistance and climate adaptability have allowed crops to grow bigger and more rapidly, but their ability to manufacture or uptake nutrients has not kept pace with their rapid growth."

Here are the specific nutrient declines: A Kushi Institute analysis of 12 fresh vegetables from 1975 to 1997 found that calcium levels dropped 27 percent, iron levels 37 percent, vitamin A levels 21 percent, and vitamin C levels 30 percent. A British study of 20 vegetables found similar declines, and another study reported that one would have to eat eight oranges today to derive the same amount of Vitamin A as our grandparents would have gotten from one.

Perhaps the new reality among such dire reports is this: supplements have become the real food – actual nutrition - and food has become the supplement. We need to restore our soils by foregoing pesticide and chemical fertilizers, and rotate crops to replenish the nutrients that are lost from industrial farming. Plants should be bred for nutritional value rather than faster yield and pesticide resistance. In the meantime, consumers will have to consider getting the body the fuel it needs by the most efficient and complete means possible – and that means supplements.

There is great resistance to fueling the body with nutritious food. Dr. Eric Braverman describes the source and scope of this resistance that is making us diseased and nonfunctional:

> *America's child knows more about Viagra than vegetables, and the average American adult will buy Viagra sooner than he buys vegetables. We have a society that has a value-structure problem. We need to reconstruct health care. We have to tackle faith, mis-trained doctors, the environment, the role of the pharmaceutical industry, the failure of education, the addiction industry's role, the lifestyle role, the hospital's role, the food industry's role, the insurance industry's role, and the clergy's failure to make an impact on anyone. - Dr. Eric Braverman*

Genetically Modified Organisms (GMO)

According to a short history, scientists first discovered, in 1946, that DNA can transfer between organisms and the first genetically modified plant or transgenic plant was produced in 1983, using an antibiotic-resistant tobacco plant. In 1994, a transgenic tomato was approved by the FDA for marketing in the U.S. - the modification allowed the tomato to delay ripening after picking. In the U.S. in 1995, an array of transgenic crops received marketing approval: canola with modified oil composition, corn/maize, cotton resistant to the herbicide bromoxynil (Calgene), Bt cotton (Monsanto), Bt potatoes (Monsanto), soybeans resistant to the herbicide glyphosate (Monsanto), virus-resistant squash (Monsanto-Asgrow), and additional delayed ripening tomatoes (DNAP, Zeneca/Peto, and Monsanto).

In 2000, with the creation of golden rice, scientists genetically modified food to increase its nutrient value for the first time. As of 2011, the U.S. leads a list of multiple countries in the production of GM crops, and 25 GM crops had received regulatory approval to be grown commercially.

As of 2013, roughly 85% of corn, 91% of soybeans, and 88% of cotton produced in the United States are genetically modified. The following chart illustrates the recent and pervasive changes that have taken place in America's food supply for a very young population.

Food	Year GMO Introduced	Percent of U.S. GMO Crops
Soy	1996	94% in 2011
Cottonseed	1996	90% in 2011
Corn	1996	88% in 2011
Canola Oil	1996	90% in 2010
Papaya	1998	80% in 2010 (Hawaii and China)
Alfalfa	2005	(cattle feed only as of 2011)
Sugar Beets	2005	90% as of 2009
Milk	1994	17% of cows injected with rBGH growth hormone as of 2007
Aspartame	1965	Found in over 6,000 products, uses GM bacteria in manufacturing

A Canadian report on the nutritional value of non-GMO corn reported the following:

Non-GMO corn contains 437 times more calcium, 56 times more magnesium, and 7 times more manganese. The GMO corn contained high levels of glyphosate and formaldehyde, both toxic to people and animals.

Baby Formula

Most baby formula is made from cow's milk, and the great majority of milk based formulas are produced from milk taken from cows injected with bovine growth hormone (rBGH), with GMO corn sweeteners added. If the baby is allergic to milk based formula, the four bestselling soy based formulas are made from genetically modified soy beans:

- Similac Soy   42%
- Gerber Good Start   48%
- Infamil   49%
- Walmart Parent's Choice   66%

The Women/Infants/Children's (WIC) program provides formula to over two million newborns in the United States. They only provide formulas containing genetically engineered soy or rBGH derived milk.

The Presence of Pesticides

Most of the genetic modifications in our food make them resistant to pesticides. The most common pesticide used in the U.S. is "RoundUp," and its active ingredient glyphosate is being detected in high levels in human beings. The German journal *Ithaca* reported that city dwellers had urine concentrations of glyphosate that were 5 to 20 times the limit for drinking water. There are few independent studies on glyphosate, because Monsanto will not allow independent research on their patented products. However, a few studies have reported birth defects in frogs and chickens, and damage to human cells. When sprayed on growing food, it becomes systemic in the food, and cannot be washed off. When eaten, it devastates the beneficial gut bacteria, compromising immunity and health. Glyphosate has been associated with endocrine disruption, reproductive issues, neurotoxicity, cancer, and DNA damage. About 180 million pounds of glyphosate were used on commercial crops as estimated by the Environmental Protection Agency in 2011. In addition 5+ million pounds were used on home gardens. Glyphosate has been detected in ground water and air samples, and does not readily break down.

Almost all corn, sugar beets, and soy are genetically modified in the United States. The changed genetic makeup of these grains resulted in altered crops that can be sprayed with specially formulated herbicides, for example "Roundup," that allows everything to die except the food crop. The take away point is that genetically modified crops are engineered to withstand extremely high levels of glyphosate, the active chemical in the herbicide, without dying along with the weeds. Glyphosate is absorbed from the soil into the plant, and then ingested by people, who suffer damage to gut flora from the glyphosate. Because it is absorbed from the soil, it can't be washed off—it's not on the food; it's in the food.

A recent report illustrates another problem that has risen from Roundup resistant food-- superweeds that are resistant to pesticides began taking hold in early 2000's. A former FDA official explains how industrial farming has dealt with superweeds: Late in 2004, weeds resistant to Monsanto's herbicide Roundup began appearing in GM plantings in Georgia and soon spread to other Southern states. By 2009, more than one hundred thousand acres in Georgia were infested with Roundup-resistant pigweed. Planters were advised to apply multiple herbicides, thereby defeating the point of Roundup: to reduce chemical applications.

Weed resistance has spread to more than 12 million U.S. acres. Many of the worst weeds, some of which grow more than six feet and can sharply reduce crop yields, have become resistant to the popular glyphosate-based weed-killer Roundup as well as other common herbicides. This is not a trivial problem. As the *Ottawa Citizen* explains, the resilience of nature is evident across almost twelve million acres of superweed-infested U.S. farmland. Some runaway weeds in the southern U.S. are said to be big enough to stop combines dead in their tracks.

The industry is pressing the U.S. and Canadian governments to approve GM corn engineered to resist 2,4-D, the principal ingredient in Agent Orange, the defoliant used during the Vietnam War. The chemical industry maintains that 2,4-D is safe at current usage levels. Maybe, but Ontario bans its use on lawns, gardens, and in school yards and parks. Weeds resistant to 2,4-D have been identified since the 1950s. Clearly if 2,4-D is going to be the "answer" to Roundup ready resistance, it will now be used in much larger quantities than in the 1950's.

A Word About Wheat—the Latest Allergy Disaster

Why is wheat absent from discussions about GMO? Sixty years ago, wheat was considered the single answer to world hunger. Strains of wheat were selectively bred, a process called hybridization, which results in the preservation of desirable traits, such as quicker maturity, more yield per acre, more calories. Wheat has been hybridized hundreds of times, and can no longer be grown in the wild. Its gluten content is so high that it causes a spike in blood sugar more drastic than eating table sugar itself! This is explained in detail in the chapter on gut health.

How to Avoid GMO Foods

Seventy percent of foods sold in the supermarket contain genetically modified ingredients. Over five million children in the United States are suffering from food allergies, a problem that correlates strongly to the development of GMO processed foods for infants and children. In spite of the complete flooding of the food market with unlabeled genetically modified food, it is relatively easy to avoid, by eliminating the following food from your family's diet:

1. Soy (tofu and soy sauce are not GMO, avoid soy lecithin)
2. Corn (all corn products, especially cereal, high fructose corn syrup and corn oil) Popcorn is not GMO
3. Canola oil and cottonseed oil (margarine, cooking oil and processed foods)

4. Sugar beets (any label that says "sugar" probably contains GMO sugar beet sugar).
5. Papaya from Hawaii and China
6. Zucchini and yellow crookneck squash
7. Beef fed with Alfalfa hay or injected with rBGH (bovine growth hormone)
8. Aspartame

Foods that are certified organic are GMO free. When I shop, I remember the four big offenders—corn, soy, sugar, and oil. I limit my oil intake to coconut oil, avocados, olive and walnut oil. These are healthy oils, and replace harmful GMO and saturated fats that are more difficult to digest. When you eliminate sugar and high fructose corn syrup, you have skipped every inside grocery aisle! Your choices become small servings of organic grass fed beef and poultry, wild caught cold water fish, and fresh or frozen organic fruits and vegetables. Thankfully eating a more clean and natural diet is not only disease preventive it is cost effective and affordable. It is time to abandon chemically treated and altered pseudo-food and re-discover the real nutrition that fuels our minds and bodies.

Choosing Food Supplements

Only protein satisfies hunger, and the key to successful and healthy food consumption is the right balance of protein, carbohydrates and healthy fats. A non-dairy (no whey) non-soy (interrupts hormone balance) vegan protein that contains a complete amino acid profile is a healthy way to curb hunger and feed the body the protein it needs. Make sure your protein is free of GM food, gluten, dairy, and soy.

Chapter 1 Recommendations:

- Avoid genetically modified foods—corn, soy, sugar beets, and canola and cottonseed oil—search labels for key words "high fructose corn syrup, lecithin, sugar, margarine, corn, soy")
- Buy grass fed beef—no alfalfa hay (GMO) or bovine growth hormone
- Eat organic poultry to avoid antibiotics
- Eliminate wheat
- Buy from local farmer's markets, or organic fruits and vegetables
- Supplement with minerals that are missing from depleted soil

Chapter 2
Hormone Balance

A Message from Deanna:

If you have ever lost control of your emotions, if for no apparent reason you have lashed out at the very people you love, if you have felt the pain and isolation of depression and chronic fatigue, or if your marriage has suffered from a libido that, well, isn't worth mentioning, then you are not alone. There are a number of indicators that your hormones are out of balance.

There is a reason why many women in the modern world feel this way, but how did this happen? And most importantly what can you do about it? These are some of the questions I hope to answer in this handbook.

As a family practice physician, I see numerous women come into the office suffering from a multitude of complaints, and traditional treatments often times provided absolutely no relief. While traditional pharmaceutical-based modern medicine can be a lifesaver in some instances, there are instances when you have to look for answers beyond the scope of that context. In my journey to find answers to pressing health problems not adequately treated within the traditional medical model, I have learned a great deal and this book contains findings and guidance that can be very helpful to many today.

I understand hormone imbalance issues after suffering from many of the symptoms listed above and more. It was not good for me, or my family. Even though I am a doctor, traditional medical approaches did not help; in fact many made me feel worse. But listen now because my story ends well.

In 2002, at the age of 33, I was practicing medicine full time, but was very sick. I had struggled with joint pain since my teenage years, often waking up and wondering if I could even walk across the floor at the age of 17. I remember thinking "What will my life be like when I am old?!" I developed other symptoms like constipation, extremely dry skin and severe fatigue, chronic abdominal pain and lethargy that led to an eventual diagnosis of hypothyroidism at the age of 18.

I married while in medical school and had my first child during my fourth year of medical school; the second child came during my internship, and my third while doing my family practice residency. I am a "type A" personality who rarely knows my own limits. I point this out because it is this personality type that can literally wake up bewildered one day in a poor state of health and wonder, "How on earth did I get here?"

After conveniently ignoring the signs my body sent all along the way and after having my third child, I ground to a halt each month with menstrual periods so heavy I thought I was having a monthly miscarriage, though I knew this was not the case. I was also occasionally experiencing moderate to severe PMS. I didn't like who I was three days out of a month and neither did my family. It was as if I had a complete personality change.

Over the next two years not only did the bleeding get worse, but I was diagnosed with psoriatic arthritis (an inflammatory type of arthritis similar to rheumatoid arthritis) by a local rheumatologist. I was told if I did not start taking a serious "disease-modifying drug" I would be in a wheelchair in 10 years time. My type-A world narrowed even further. Delivering that diagnosis to me - a person who hit the floor running first thing in the morning and who continued in this mode all day until she fell into bed - was like issuing a death sentence.

Reluctantly, I started the medication. A medication injected weekly with numerous side effects. While the arthritis pain improved, everything else seemed to deteriorate. The most serious side effect of this medication was that it completely wiped out my immune system. I caught every cold, flu and strep throat that came my way and I had developed some pretty severe gastrointestinal problems.

During this time, a close friend and patient, who knew of my heavy periods gave me a bioidentical progesterone cream. My bleeding was so severe by this time, I was anemic. To manage my growing health issues, I often had to cancel patients because I felt terrible. I tried everything conventional medicine and my profession had to offer and was ready to have a hysterectomy.

Not hoping for much I looked at the bioidentical progesterone given to me by a non-medical friend and I decided I didn't have anything to lose so I tried it, applying it to my skin for transdermal absorption. To my amazement, it worked very well. In fact, I could tell a difference at my next cycle! After using it for three months, my periods became normal and my PMS went away completely! From the time I started my period as a teen, I had always determined when my period would start based upon how I felt. It was the only time that I was ever grumpy.

I retested my blood work after three months of this progesterone therapy to find that my anemia had been resolved and my thyroid function had improved. Why didn't I know about this? Why isn't this being taught in medical schools? It's such an inexpensive and easy solution to so many women's issues. That experience began my personal education and relentless pursuit to find out everything I possibly could about bioidentical progesterone and its therapeutic uses. I was amazed at what I learned. This experience opened my mind to a different approach to medicine. It gave me permission, in a sense, to start thinking outside of the box, to start looking at health from a different perspective: To start looking for the root cause of the problem and not just treating symptoms with a medication.

I was suffering from a pretty severe hormone imbalance called estrogen dominance/progesterone deficiency. It didn't happen overnight, but instead was a gradual process, an incremental decline in my overall health. The ending to my story is very positive. I learned the absolute importance of proper diet, of using dietary supplements, and of the benefits of many herbs. I was able to see my hormones come into balance, my arthritis and GI issues resolve through the use of these supplements and herbs, and my overall health improved tremendously. As my health improved, I related my journey of recovery to the women in our medical practice. There were so many women coming for PMS, depression, decreased sex drive, and so much more. Many patients unquestioningly rely upon birth control. However, women of all ages - from teenagers to postmenopausal - may not fully understand the potential for negative outcomes associated with birth control use.

For example, there are many 30-40-somethings I have treated who experience classic symptoms related to their history of birth control pill use. The domino effect can look something like this: after taking birth control, migraine headaches can develop, then migraine medication is added to the birth control. Patients can become depressed from the effects of the birth control's high estrogen exposure, leading to a prescription for antidepressants. (I specifically remember being told by a psychiatrist, during one of my psychiatry rotations, that many mental illnesses would go away or be less complicated, if I could get people off of birth control pills. This was especially true among adolescents.) At this point, a patient may find they have absolutely no interest in sex. Often they gain weight, especially around the mid-section due to the estrogen they are ingesting via birth control. In addition, cravings for carbohydrates and refined sugars can become seemingly uncontrollable and lead to increased weight gain and high insulin levels. Due to the additional weight and chronically high levels of circulating insulin, patients can become insulin resistant and be at risk for diabetes and high blood pressure, both of which require treatment with more medications. At this point, in what is a relatively short period of time, the patient often feels terrible; she's overweight, depressed, has migraines, no interest in sex, has been diagnosed with diabetes and hypertension, and is taking, on average, 5-9 medications! Sound familiar? It's then that she wakes up and says, "How did I get here?" Usually it is a process so gradual that she hardly noticed. Is that the track that you are on? Or is that the track someone you know and care very much about is on?

We have access to so much more information than our parents and grandparents. The New England Journal of Medicine states that "Preventable illness makes up approximately 70 percent of the burden of disease and the associated costs." There are many great resources available to educate yourself and take control of your own health and wellness. You won't learn everything overnight. It is a gradual process to return to health naturally. But, my promise to you is that you can begin to feel better in a week's time. Today I am in great health and you can be too.

Dr. Deanna

Hormone Imbalance

Hormone imbalance is a condition that may affect a woman early, even at the onset of menses. Years ago the average age girls started their periods was about 16, but currently the average age at the onset of menstruation is around 12. Exposure to environmental estrogens and the increasing amount of body fat in young adults is believed to play a role in this change. Body fat on its own produces estrogens and may increase the levels of these hormones circulating in the bloodstream.

Today over 50 percent of adolescent females experience some menstrual dysfunction. This may include dysfunctional uterine bleeding (abnormal menstruation either in the amount of bleeding or the frequency), amenorrhea (no menstruation), dysmenorrhea (painful menstruation), and premenstrual syndrome (PMS). Most PMS is minor, mild cramping and pain with minor variations in cycles. However, in some cases it can be severe and includes debilitating dysmenorrhea and severe abnormal uterine bleeding. In some cases, the bleeding may cause significant anemia from blood loss. About 45-70 percent of all post-pubescent females have some degree of dysmenorrhea, with up to 15 percent of these females describing the pain as severe and being incapacitated for 1-3 days per month.

Hormonal imbalance affects 80 percent of U.S. women at peri-menopause (the time period before the cessation of the menstrual cycle, sometimes beginning as early as thirty-five years of age) when disruptive and persistent symptoms can appear. This can be very frustrating for a woman with this condition and also for her immediate family, her doctor and even her employer. Most women have an idea the symptoms they are experiencing seem to have a hormonal component because the symptoms often worsen with their menstrual cycle, but they don't know what to do about this condition, and quite honestly, most physicians do not know what to do with them either. Due to widespread misunderstanding, it is not uncommon for these women to be placed on birth control pills or antidepressant therapies, which in the long run, can make the problem worse.

Some of the symptoms of hormonal imbalance are stress, acne, menstrual cramps, hair loss, PMS, fatigue, irritability, hot flashes, night sweats, migraine headaches, endometriosis, infertility, decreased sex drive, depression, weight gain, osteoporosis or osteopenia, dry skin, polycystic ovarian syndrome (PCOS), abnormal periods, heavy or painful periods, first trimester miscarriages, joint pain and breast cancer. Sounds like a lot of people you know, doesn't it? Hormone imbalance is a condition that has reached epidemic proportions.

Our bodies are very complex and the reproductive hormones are a central part of the mix! Women have many hormones that affect their reproduction, but the focus of this section of the handbook is primarily on estrogen and progesterone. No discussion of reproductive hormones would be complete however without mentioning the adrenal hormones and thyroid hormones, so included at the end of this handbook is a brief section on adrenal glands and thyroid hormones.

How Two Sex Hormones Work

Estrogen and progesterone are sex hormones made primarily in the ovaries. They work together so that a woman is able to have children, but when these two are out of balance, the result can affect not only health, but wellbeing. Estrogen is the hormone that is most active during the first half of a woman's cycle. It is responsible for development of the egg and development of the lining of the uterus. At about the 14th day of a woman's cycle ovulation occurs. This is also when a woman will have an increase in progesterone levels. The mature egg has been released and the remnant of the egg, the corpus luteum, signals the brain causing progesterone to be produced, largely in the ovaries.

Progesterone is the pregnancy hormone, because a woman cannot maintain a pregnancy without it, but progesterone deficiencies can be harmful to women. If progesterone is deficient, a woman will not be able to maintain the endometrial lining or the fertilized egg. This deficiency is the most common cause of first trimester miscarriages. Progesterone is highly active in the 2nd half of the woman's cycle. It is responsible for maintaining the lining of the uterus so that the egg can implant. Progesterone has an opposing or "balancing" effect on estrogen, sending the message that the endometrial lining can stop growing because it is sufficient for implantation of the egg.

It is during the 2nd trimester of pregnancy, after the 3rd month, that the placenta surrounding the baby is developed and takes over the function of progesterone production. During the last trimester of pregnancy the placenta will produce up to 400mg of progesterone a day. The average non-pregnant female only makes about 20mg per day. In addition to its important reproductive aspects, progesterone is an important hormone in the fetal development of the central nervous system, including the brain. There are some recent studies that link progesterone to the development or repair of nerves. Nerves are wrapped with a coating called myelin sheath. The myelin sheath is made up of cells called Schwann cells. It appears that progesterone stimulates the production of these Schwann cells. Given that the body was created with the amazing ability to repair or heal itself, it is reasonable to conclude that the stimulation/production of Schwann cells by progesterone is the body's attempt to repair neurological damage.

It is very important for any woman considering the use of bioidentical hormones to maintain or achieve balance in her life to know or learn how her body works. Our bodies send many "signals" which can be recognized, if we pay attention, but most of us either don't see the signals or don't understand what our bodies are saying to us. Since hormones fluctuate minute by minute in our system based upon stress, emotion, physical condition, etc., it is important that we learn to recognize those signals and respond appropriately. For example, there are times when a woman's body may only need to be supplemented with 20mg of USP Progesterone and there are stressful times when she will need 40mg of USP Progesterone per day. The woman who is tuned in and listening to her body can recognize the signals more effectively and better manage hormonal imbalances. The doctor's advice is that you need to know your body better than anyone else.

It is important to realize that, while the focus here is primarily on the use of bioidentical USP Progesterone, there are often cases in which a woman is not only low in progesterone but also in estrogen. In that case, transdermal (applied to the skin) estrogen can be used. I have used transdermal Bioidentical estrogen in my practice in the form of Bi-est, which is a combination of estradiol and estriol. These are two of the three forms of estrogen and are often referred to in literature as E1 and E3.

Estriol is the estrogen a woman makes during pregnancy and is the safest of the estrogens. Some studies show that it is actually estrogen metabolites that seem to stimulate cancer cells, not the estrogen. In a sense, estriol is like a saturated fat. It cannot be oxidized into a metabolite making it a safer estrogen to supplement. Estrone is the strongest estrogen and potentially the most harmful. The subject of which estrogen to take is certainly an important

one, but not one covered in this handbook, but know this - estrogen should NEVER be taken by mouth, even if it is a bioidentical estrogen. The reason estrogen should not be taken by mouth is that as it passes through the liver it is metabolized into the more dangerous form of estrogen, estrone.

Hormones get out of balance through a variety of factors including dietary consumption of estrogens, lifestyle, medications, and even environment. Diet plays a big role. A diet high in carbohydrates or simple sugars will make hormonal imbalance worse. When you are consuming a diet high in carbohydrates your body's response is to have high circulating insulin levels. High insulin levels can be deleterious because insulin is a growth hormone and it is the only hormone in the body that causes us to store fat in fat cells. Estrogen can be made in fat cells. A high carbohydrate diet will make you pack on weight around the waist, in particular, further contributing to hormone imbalance.

Life style is another big factor. Most of us are constantly on the go, trying feverishly to meet deadlines, pick up kids, run errands, and literally hold it all together! A person under a lot of stress will generally produce a lot of cortisol hormone made by the adrenal glands. One of the building blocks of cortisol is progesterone. If you allow yourself to remain in a constant state of stress requiring high levels of cortisol, it can force your body to use up progesterone stores to make cortisol. Important to note is that the body's hormones are all interrelated and best work in a symphony all balanced together.[3]

High levels of cortisol are particularly deleterious to you, because over time it will interfere with your sleep cycles, shut down your immune system, and give you a significantly higher risk for developing cancer. This cycle is very taxing to the adrenal glands because this is where cortisol is made and will eventually lead to adrenal fatigue and/or failure.

Medications play a role in hormone imbalance, as some can wrongly bind to our body's natural hormone receptors, and block access of our beneficial hormones. Birth control pills and synthetic hormone replacement therapy (traditional hormone replacement therapy HRT) play a huge role in blocking hormone receptors.

On the other end of the reproductive cycle, sadly, many adolescents are prescribed birth control pills to control acne, treat PMS, to decrease amounts of bleeding during the menstrual cycle, to prevent pregnancy and even for the sake of convenience. Many are now given what is called "continuous birth control" which stops the menstrual cycle for a year. This is a very dangerous! Birth control pills completely control hormonal cycles with man-made hormones, shutting down a woman's natural hormone production. Use of birth control pills is linked to breast cancer, and the longer a woman takes them the greater her risk. We are at an unprecedented time in medicine where many women start birth control at the age of 14, take it through their childbearing years, and then transition to hormone replacement therapy in their menopausal years. Since the 1970s, many women have consumed artificial hormones for 30 years or more! Never has the use of synthetic hormones for this length of time been studied.

In August, 2005, the World Health Organization's International Agency for Research on Cancer issued a little publicized statement reclassifying chemical birth control as a Group 1 carcinogenic, the highest classification of carcinogenicity given by the research group. The researchers included 21 scientists from 8 countries, and they concluded that oral contraceptives increase the risk of breast, cervix, and liver cancer. The study was reported in the British Medical Journal, *The Lancet*, which stated that more than 100 million women—about 10% of all women of reproductive age worldwide—use combined oral contraceptives, and use is rising.

Dr. Schwarzbein explains an important distinction between our bodies' hormones and chemical substances formulated to replace them:

> *Birth control pills are not hormones; they are drugs that disrupt a woman's sex hormone balance. Since all of the hormones of the body are connected, BCP's affect all your hormone systems. The longer you take BCP's the greater your hormonal imbalances.*

If you are the mother of a young daughter, I appeal to you to do some research of your own into the risks associated with birth control before walking this path with your adolescent. My advice is the risks are simply not worth it. Synthetic hormones are fakes. They are man-made attempts to mimic Mother Nature, which simply cannot be done.

Physicians have been taught in medical schools, since the turn of the century, that natural functions of a woman's body including menses, pregnancy, child birth, and menopause are diseases to be treated by drug intervention. These chemicals have caused profound disruption in body hormone balance resulting in chronic illnesses and life threatening cancers. In spite of this potentially dire risk, the medical establishment views birth control as vital to our lives and an integral part of our culture. As evolutionary beings, youth are no longer considered capable of self-control; therefore pregnancy cannot be avoided without the aid of birth control, and is necessary to prevent unwanted pregnancy in spite of its accompanying lethal side effects. Breast cancer is a small price to pay for sexual liberation, according to the prevailing public health model.

Somewhere in the process, women have been reduced from mothers and daughters making decisions for their good health, to statistics as a dot on the population scatter chart. However, scatter charts don't measure the grief and tragedy of reproductive disease so personal to each life touched by the disfigurement and death. The facts must be known, so we can make intelligent and informed decisions based on individual good health, and for the future of our children and grandchildren.

HORMONE BALANCE TEST

Symptoms: (Progesterone Deficiency)	Symptoms: (Estrogen Deficiency)	Symptoms: (DHEA)
❑ Large breasts ❑ Swollen tender and painful breasts ❑ Edema/swelling ❑ Irritable and aggressive ❑ Heavy periods ❑ Painful periods ❑ PMS ❑ Insomnia ❑ Cyclical headaches ❑ Infertility ❑ Early miscarriage ❑ Migraines ❑ Anxious/depressed	❑ Vaginal dryness ❑ Painful intercourse ❑ Bladder infections ❑ Hot flashes ❑ Night sweats ❑ Memory problems ❑ Lethargic ❑ Depression ❑ Hair loss on the top of the head ❑ Vertical wrinkles above lip ❑ Droopy breasts ❑ Hairy face	❑ Dry hair ❑ Dry skin ❑ Flabby muscles ❑ Fat belly ❑ Scant underarm hair ❑ Scant pubic hair ❑ Low libido ❑ Prone to high blood pressure, atherosclerosis, heart disease ❑ Poor immunity, cancer, infections ❑ Hard climbing stairs when over 65 years old ❑ Insecure, anxious, gloomy and sad
Symptoms: (Growth Hormone Deficiency)	**Symptoms: (Excessive Estrogen)**	**Symptoms: (Aldosterone)**
❑ Thinning hair ❑ Sagging cheeks ❑ Flabby abdomen ❑ Dry and thin skin ❑ Feeling exhausted ❑ Large wrinkles on face ❑ Forehead creases ❑ Double chin	❑ Hair loss ❑ Prostate enlargement ❑ Irritability ❑ Puffiness/bloating ❑ Headaches ❑ Breast enlargement ❑ Weight gain	❑ Low blood pressure ❑ Dizzy when standing up ❑ Feel better lying down ❑ Crave salty food ❑ Frequent urination ❑ Dehydrated skin
Symptoms: (Excessive Androgens- male hormones)	**Symptoms: (Testosterone deficiency – men & women)**	**Symptoms: (Cortisol deficiency)**
❑ Acne ❑ Excessive hair on the face and arms ❑ Thinning hair on the head ❑ Ovarian cysts ❑ Polycystic ovarian syndrome (PCOS) ❑ Hypoglycemia and/or unstable blood sugar ❑ Infertility ❑ Mid cycle pain	❑ Weight loss ❑ Loss of muscle ❑ Lower sex drive ❑ Constant fatigue ❑ Enlarged breasts ❑ Lower stamina ❑ Softer erections (male) ❑ Gallbladder problems ❑ Tire easily with exercise ❑ Fat belly ❑ Slack & wrinkled face ❑ Constantly depressed	❑ Debilitating fatigue ❑ Foggy thinking ❑ Thin and/or dry skin ❑ Brown spots on face ❑ Unstable blood sugar ❑ Low blood pressure ❑ Intolerance to exercise ❑ Crave salt & sugar ❑ Allergies weak & trembly after stress
Symptoms: (Thyroid Deficiency)		
❑ Cold sensitivity ❑ Cold extremities ❑ Easy weight gain ❑ Dry skin ❑ Hair loss ❑ More tired in the morning ❑ Constipated	❑ Puffy face and eyelids in morning ❑ Slow and unclear thinking ❑ Prone to skin cancers ❑ Dry lusterless, thick hair ❑ Big calves ❑ More tired after napping or resting	❑ Morning leg and ankle swelling ❑ Pear shaped trunk, padded buttocks and thighs ❑ Depressed in the morning ❑ Elevated diastolic blood pressure ❑ Joint stiffness in the morning

Chart: Dr. Allan Lieberman, MD. Center for Occupational & Environmental Medicine. Chareslton, SC. www.coem.com.

Many people do not realize that hormones in pills, patches and vaginal rings are being excreted in an active form in the urine of the women taking them. Those active forms make it to the waterways and eventually back to us. Along the way they cause significant reproductive changes to fish and other creatures living in our waterways. There are many studies that show 30 percent of male fish in lakes and rivers in the U.S. produce eggs like a female. The scientists studying fish attribute this reproductive confusion to the estrogens humans excrete into the waterways. This issue should be of great concern. Tighter regulations on these medications and better water treatment strategies are needed, or we can expect similar changes among our own species. It may not be as drastic as male animals producing eggs, but certainly decreased sperm counts in humans found by researchers today are being attributed to this cause. The research is well documented and yet it seems to get little attention from our government and the media. Pharmaceutical and chemical companies have very deep pockets, which can cause watchdog agencies to turn a blind eye to these problems.

I cannot overlook the impact that our environment has on the issue of hormone imbalance. There are many chemicals in our environment that have the ability to bind to estrogen receptors and create an unwanted effect in the body, such as pesticides, plastics, household cleaning products, cosmetic products that are petroleum-based or that contain mineral oil, herbicides, fungicides and the list continues. These compounds that are able to bind to receptors and interfere with our natural hormones are often referred to as xenoestrogens or "false estrogen." To say that we are swimming in a sea of estrogen would be a very accurate description!

The Difference Between Bioidentical Hormones and Synthetic Hormones

The difference between the way synthetic hormones and bioidentical hormones work in the body is like the difference between night and day! A synthetic hormone is a man-made version, or copycat of what the body makes, but not exactly. While the synthetic version may have some of the same effects as the "real deal", it comes with many adverse side effects.

The biochemical and molecular composition of a bioidentical hormone is identical to that which our bodies make, so the phrase bioidentical USP Progesterone, refers to progesterone hormone exactly like our body makes on its own. A great deal of the confusion in this matter exists because of the confusion in the medical field. My experience in medical school was the difference between bioidentical and non-bioidentical was simply not taught. Progesterone is viewed as the same thing as progestin (the term for the pharmaceutical version). It is wrong to view them as the same because the chemical composition is so different! Progesterone actually is breast protective as well as supporting and maintaining pregnancy. However, synthetic progestins are indicated in breast cancer and absolutely contraindicated during pregnancy and may cause serious birth defects. Quite a difference!

Progesterone Supplements

To use progesterone properly, it is important to understand how a woman's cycle works. The average woman will have a 28-day menstrual cycle, but most women are not average and will find that their actual cycle is a little shorter or a little longer. In a 28-day cycle, day 1 of the cycle is the day you start to bleed. Day 14 is when you ovulate and then day 28 is the day before you start your period. The only thing that is consistent in a woman's cycle is that 14 days after she ovulates, if she is not pregnant, she will start to menstruate.

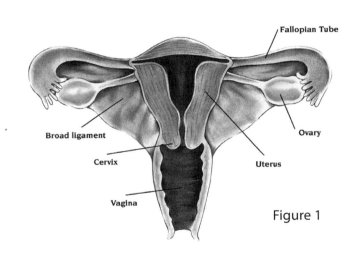

Fallopian Tube
Broad ligament
Cervix
Ovary
Uterus
Vagina

Figure 1

When a woman ovulates is often the tricky part. For some it is on day 8; for others it might be day 16! When ovulation occurs there is a peak in progesterone levels. It appears that this peak is in part responsible for the woman's increased sex drive during ovulation. Some women will feel a slight cramping low in the abdomen associated with ovulation. Most women will experience a slight discharge that is clear, stringy and odorless. The clear, stringy nature of the discharge is often described as having an egg white-like consistency. After ovulation the egg makes its way to the fallopian tube (see figure 1) where it may or may not be fertilized. If it is fertilized, the egg will implant into the woman's uterine lining where it will start to grow and develop. If the egg is not fertilized, the endometrial lining of the uterus starts to slough off, which is the start of the woman's period. Over and over and over this process repeats 12 times a year, or, on average, 444 times during her reproductive life! All womenneed to read and learn about how their bodies work. Investigating fertility awareness is one way to begin your learning curve.

Evaluating a Progesterone Product

There are a few things that are important to look for in finding a progesterone product. It is important to find progesterone that is bioidentical and USP Progesterone, which means it meets high United States Pharmacopeia standards. Bioidentical simply means that one molecule of progesterone from the product would look exactly like a molecule of progesterone made in a woman's body. USP guarantees that you are actually getting progesterone and not just a soy cream or a wild yam cream. The product should be in an airtight container, so that it is not being continually oxidized by exposure to the air. Avoid using progesterone that comes in a jar, because scooping out the product by hand can contaminate it. You should also look at the base ingredients with which the progesterone was mixed, to make sure that there is no mineral oil. Mineral oil can interfere with the body's ability to appropriately absorb progesterone. It's also a petrochemical and I do not recommend using skin care products that contain it. USP Progesterone is readily available within the marketplace and can easily be obtained through a local health food store, compounding pharmacy, or health and wellness company.

Hormone Testing

It is important to understand that in many cases hormones being tested in the venous blood do not give a true picture of what is going on in the body. A vast majority (up to 99 percent) of the sex hormones are carried in the blood via sex hormone binding globulin (SHBG). This is the inactive (storage) form of the sex hormones. The free hormone which is not bound to the SHBG is the active form. It is bound to fatty substances because it is totally insoluble in water. This active form is not measured in the serum because the fatty substances are "spun off" in the centrifuge in processing the blood for testing. The best way to test hormones is either through a saliva test or through a "blood spot" test. The free active form of sex hormones is easily tested in a saliva test or a peripheral tissue "blood spot" test via a finger prick. Saliva and blood spot testing are dependable and are becoming more widely used. You can order a saliva test or blood spot test online through ZRT labs in Beaverton, Oregon (www.ZRTlabs.com). Saliva testing is great for checking hormone levels as well as cortisol levels. The blood spot can be used to check hormone levels, thyroid levels, insulin levels, Vitamin D levels and much more.

Hormone Issues and Progesterone Guidelines

Using Progesterone for Endometriosis

Endometriosis is a painful female condition that can have a negative impact on one's ability to become pregnant. It can cause heavy and painful periods as well. The exact cause of endometriosis is unknown but what happens in this disease is that pieces of the endometrial lining (lining of the uterus) are outside of the uterus. The pieces are often called "endometrial implants" and they may attach themselves to the inside of the abdomen, the ovaries, the colon and even the fallopian tubes. Most women experience severe cramping with their period when they have endometriosis.

Studies suggest that endometriosis is related to environmental artificial estrogens. Dr. Elizabeth Smith cites studies conducted by the Canadian government on exposure to xenoestrogens (synthetic chemicals that mimic estrogen in the body) and the resulting endometriosis. She writes,

> It is likely that xenoestrogens, chemicals that mimick estrogen, are causing the epidemic of endometriosis that we are seeing in young women. Gerhard and Runnebaum (1992) first brought attention to the link between the high levels of dioxins in blood and endometriosis. Scientific research with female rhesus monkeys fed different amounts of dioxin-laden foods supports epidemiological studies, suggesting that endometriosis in humans is caused by xenohormones (foreign hormones).

Another clue that endometriosis is related to hormone balance is its connection to autoimmune diseases. Author and researcher Mary Shomon reports that as many as 12 percent of women with endometriosis had lupus or multiple sclerosis, vs. 2 percent in the general population, and 42 percent of these women had under-active thyroid glands, versus approximately 5 percent of the general population.

One thing certain is that endometriosis was never described before the industrial/petrochemical age. Endometriosis is very debilitating and painful, and would not have escaped the scrutiny of physicians of the pre-industrial age. Thirty to fifty percent of women with endometriosis are infertile, and are predisposed to certain cancers, particularly early-onset breast and ovarian cancers, non-Hodgkin's lymphomas, and melanoma; as well as autoimmune diseases (in which the body attacks its own cells), such as systemic lupus erythematosus, hypothyroidism, rheumatoid arthritis, and multiple sclerosis.

Ironically, most physicians treat endometriosis with oral contraceptives, thus introducing synthetic estrogens to the body that may already be overloaded with chemicals that mimic our natural estrogen. In the short term, it relieves symptoms, because the lining of the uterus does not go through the natural process of thickening and sloughing. Some doctors recommend continuous estrogen which eliminates altogether the monthly sloughing of the uterine lining during menstruation. Twenty years ago, endometriosis almost always led to hysterectomy, the number one operation in the United States in 1980.

I recommend patients use 20-30mg of USP Progesterone daily for endometriosis. It is best to break the dose in half and use 10mg in the morning and 10-20mg in the evening. I also recommend using it all month long except when menstruating. It is best to follow these guidelines for about 3-4 months. At that time, if the woman is doing better and noticing a decrease in symptoms, I recommend that she start using progesterone at ovulation or on days 12-26 of her cycle (this is assuming she has a normal 28-day cycle).

PCOS (Polycystic Ovarian Syndrome) or PCOD (Polycystic Ovarian Disease)

PCOS is a condition that affects the ovaries with the development of multiple cysts on the ovaries. The ovaries become diseased and infertility may become an issue. There is a metabolic component to PCOS as well. High levels of carbohydrates and simple sugars stimulate the body to produce high levels of insulin. Insulin will stimulate the production of androgens (male hormones). Many of these women will also suffer from facial hair and acne due to the excessive male hormones often produced. It is commonplace to treat PCOS with oral diabetic medications to reduce the levels of insulin. It would be much wiser and safer to treat the problem through strict diet, eliminating simple carbs and refined sugars, and supplementing with progesterone. I recommend patients use 20-30mg USP progesterone daily for 90 days. Stop after 90 days and menstruation should occur. Start using 20mg daily on days 12-26 of the menstrual cycle. At this point women should be having regular periods. Many women with PCOS who are trying to get pregnant can conceive as early as month 4.

Using Progesterone for PMS

PMS can be a debilitating condition for so many women and those around them. It is surprising how common the problem is and I believe it has much to do with excess estrogen in the environment to which women are exposed. Too often antidepressants are the therapeutic response used by traditional medicine. Sometimes antidepressants are prescribed for the entire month and sometimes only prescribed for the week of

PMS. The problem with antidepressants is the lengthy side effect profile that can lead to the use of additional medications. I recommend patients use 20-30mg of USP Progesterone for the treatment of PMS. Progesterone will mainly address the mood swings, irritability and anxiety associated with PMS. Most women find progesterone works well for them when they use it on days 12-26 of their cycle, just before ovulation. For example, women who ovulate earlier than day 14 of their cycle, may want to start using it 2 days prior to ovulation. For a woman who normally ovulates on day 10, she should start using progesterone on day 8. This form of progesterone dosing is referred to as cyclical because it is designed to mimic what your body does naturally.

Using Progesterone for Abnormal Bleeding

Abnormal bleeding requires some special considerations. Any woman experiencing abnormal uterine bleeding (sometimes called dysfunctional uterine bleeding) should see a doctor first before trying progesterone. Although this is a very common problem due to hormonal imbalance, abnormal bleeding can also be a sign of endometrial cancer. Once endometrial cancer has been ruled out, then 20-30mg USP Progesterone can be used on days 12-26 of the menstrual cycle.

Using Progesterone for First Trimester Miscarriage

If you have suffered from a first trimester miscarriage or know a woman who has, you know how devastating it can be. Many women are plagued with multiple first trimester miscarriages due to a low progesterone level. Please read the previous section on progesterone use for infertility. If you have had a first trimester miscarriage in the past and want to use progesterone in an attempt to prevent it from happening again, I recommend using 40-60mg of transdermal USP Progesterone daily, the moment you find out you are pregnant. If you are already using progesterone when you get pregnant it is best to increase it to the 60mg daily, if you have a history of first trimester miscarriages. It is not necessary to use transdermal progesterone for the entire pregnancy. At about the 16th week of pregnancy the placenta starts to produce large quantities of progesterone. It is acceptable at this point to stop using the transdermal progesterone. By the last trimester the placenta produces up to 400mg of progesterone a day! Remember this hormone is not only critical to maintain a pregnancy, but it is also very important in the development of the baby's central nervous system.

Using Progesterone for Osteopenia or Osteoporosis

Many women have bone loss over time without even realizing it and can greatly suffer with the results. The healthcare statistics on dollars spent treating osteoporosis and the subsequent effects are staggering. Estrogen is often prescribed for this condition, but it only stops bone loss. The good news is progesterone actually stimulates osteoblasts, cells within the bone that build bone. Many women using progesterone therapy will see improvements in their bone density tests over time. To maintain bone health, I recommend 10mg USP Progesterone topically per day.

Using Progesterone for Postpartum Depression

Postpartum depression can be a serious condition with life-threatening consequences for mother and baby. Women with PMS have a higher risk of developing postpartum depression. Progesterone is safe for use in the postpartum period and while breastfeeding. I have witnessed 20mg of transdermal USP Progesterone daily applied at night to be effective in the treatment of postpartum depression. Since progesterone has a calming effect it naturally helps with insomnia and anxiety as well.

Using Progesterone for Depression, Anxiety and Insomnia

Many women in the U.S. have been improperly placed on antidepressant therapies when actually the root cause of their problem is hormone imbalance. When depression gets worse during the menstrual cycle or just before the cycle begins, it is a strong indication that a hormonal component exists. I recommend using 20mg of transdermal USP Progesterone daily. It is best used at night because it can help with sleep issues. An additional 10 to 20mg of progesterone can be used anytime during the day to treat anxiety.

Antidepressants are a multimillion-dollar industry, and their manufacturers fund research, conferences, speakers, and distributors to widen the uses for their product. After huge problems with the Women's Health Initiative became public, women were anxious to get off synthetic hormones, and to remedy emotional consequences of hormone imbalance. Antidepressants were promoted by pharmaceutical companies as a safe substitute. Antidepressants can decrease serotonin levels over time, causing a disruption of endocrine balance compounding emotional disturbance, which patients probably do not understand.

Antidepressants now carry a warning because of their association with violence and suicide. The S.A.V.E. project has collected almost 5,000 media articles identifying a violent act by someone taking antidepressants, including more than 60 school rampages by teens killing unarmed children. A 2010 peer reviewed study identified 1,527 cases of violence from FDA adverse drug reports from 31 drugs over a five year period, 2004 to 2009. They report,

> *Acts of violence towards others are a genuine and serious adverse drug event associated with a relatively small group of drugs. Varenicline, which increases the availability of dopamine, and antidepressants with serotonergic effects were the most strongly and consistently implicated drugs.*

According to the Surgeon General's report on mental health, the prevailing hypothesis for the cause of depression is depletion of both serotonin and catecholamines in the brain. If a woman's serotonin levels are depleted due to hormone imbalance, she may present to her doctor with symptoms of depression, for which she is prescribed an antidepressant. However, this acts to prevent the reuptake of serotonin, and the body will shift its production to lower levels of serotonin to compensate; then the lower levels of serotonin exacerbate the depletion, and the depression can become worse over the long term. The vicious cycle of hormone imbalance induced by chemical birth control and treatment by antidepressants, which further decreases serotonin levels, will continue until the root cause for the serotonin imbalance is addressed. To illustrate how complicated this can be, and how hormones act upon each other to balance the body, Pat Rackowski, a patient advocate treating thyroid disease writes,

> *Treating women with PMS with anti-depressants, and likewise treating women with cyclical migraine headaches with Imitrex or other migraine medicines, only covers up a problem of hormone imbalance, if it even works. Sometimes these problems are caused by serotonin deficiencies or irregularities, but the production of serotonin itself is subject to thyroid sufficiency. Thyroid is a more basic hormone than estrogen and progesterone in the sense that proper functioning of the ovaries is dependent upon thyroid.*
>
> *The same goes for proper functioning of the brain and the production of neurotransmitters such as serotonin.*

Dr. Eric Braverman, a neurological integrative medicine specialist who practices in New York, has developed a test for determining your neurological health. The Braverman Assessment, which is available online for free at http://www.forresthealth. com/forms/braverman1.pdf, is a helpful instrument to identify the body's deficiencies and imbalances which are the root cause of depression. At the end of the assessment, a specific supplement regimen is recommended for identified deficiencies of dopamine, acetylcholine, GABA, and serotonin.

Progesterone can also be used in conjunction with antidepressant therapy. Many women want to get off their antidepressant medication, but this always needs to be done with the assistance of their physician. I usually have them start using the progesterone and reevaluate their depressive symptoms 2-3 months later. At that point, if doing well, I would consider tapering off their antidepressant medication.

Using Progesterone for Decreased Libido or Low Sex Drive

Often women on progesterone therapy will notice an increase in sex drive. This is because their hormones come back into balance with the addition of progesterone allowing their body to make a small amount of testosterone through one of the many biochemical hormonal pathways. Testosterone works to increase sex drive and progesterone can help to balance the adrenals, if there is adrenal fatigue. Reducing mental and physical stress on the body is critical to overall health and reducing stress. Adrenal fatigue can itself cause a decrease in sex drive.

Permanent Loss of Sex Drive

With mounting anecdotal evidence of loss of libido in otherwise healthy young women, the effects of oral contraceptives may provide scientific support for this decrease in normal function and may demonstrate censorship operating in the U.S., related to findings of negative side effects. One prominent Boston researcher's findings reported only in England describes how oral contraceptives curb the production of testosterone, which governs sex drive in both men and women. The testosterone level is curbed by the production of sex hormone binding globulin (SHBG), which ties up testosterone and blocks its effects.

Dr. Irwin Goldstein, founder of the Institute for Sexual Medicine at the University of Boston, studied 125 women attending a sexual dysfunction clinic, and found that those who had stopped taking the pill still had an SHBG level three to four times higher than those who had never used the pill. Dr. Goldstein reported, "There's a possibility it is imprinting a woman for the rest of her life."

Using progesterone for menopausal symptoms

Many women who were on synthetic HRT (Hormone Replacement Therapy) wanted to discontinue it after the important Women's Health Initiative study results were released in 2002. The Women's Health Initiative study reported that using synthetic estrogens and progestins lead to an increase in stroke, heart attack and breast cancer. The FDA recommends that if a woman is prescribed HRT it should be for the shortest time period possible. I also know that the combination of non-bioidentical estrogen and progestin absolutely increases one's risk of developing dementia and lung cancer.

I have had good results helping women cope with menopausal symptoms and titrating off of HRT with the use of bioidentical USP Progesterone. Progesterone can help with many menopausal symptoms. Specifically it can relieve hot flashes, vaginal dryness, mood swings, and irritability. It is the sudden decrease in estrogen that causes a woman to experience hot flashes or night sweats. A woman's body can use progesterone to produce a small amount of estrogen, if the body needs it. Helene Leonetti, M.D., in a double-blind study of progesterone cream that was published in the journal, *Obstetrics and Gynecology* in 1999, showed that menopausal symptoms such as hot flashes responded very nicely to progesterone cream in 83 percent of the women, while only 19 percent of women using the placebo got relief.[4]

Progesterone as an Alternative to HRT

If a woman is currently on an HRT and wants to get off of it, I recommend using 20-30 mg of progesterone daily for a month in addition to her HRT. In the second month cut the pill in half while continuing with the transdermal progesterone. In month 3, decrease the HRT pill to 1/2 a pill every other day while using the progesterone and then discontinue the HRT in month 4. During this entire time, use 20mg-30mg of transdermal USP Progesterone, all month with a 5 day break each month.

There are some progesterone products that include phytoestrogens or plant estrogens that can also be beneficial in resolving hot flashes. It is of benefit to take the 5 day break each month in an attempt to let the progesterone receptor sites down regulate or clear out. This will allow the product to work at a higher efficacy. Many women, after hearing about the WHI, stopped taking their Premarin or Prempro cold turkey. Many were miserable in doing this and suffered severe hot flashes and other symptoms. This is not necessary and can be avoided if the woman tapers off of her HRT and supplements with bioidentical progesterone. If a woman gets good results with this approach I usually recommend that she continue using the progesterone. If she is using a product with plant estrogens and is doing fine in terms of symptoms a year later, she can switch to using USP Progesterone without phytoestrogens.

Neurological Symptoms Related to Hormone Imbalance

The *Journal of the American Medical Association* [JAMA] reported, based on the Women's Health Initiative data, there is an increased risk of Alzheimer's disease, as well as milder forms of dementia for women taking synthetic hormones. Dr. Sally Shumaker of Wake Forest University reported that synthetic estrogen users face a 38 percent increased risk of developing dementia or forgetfulness. On February 10, 2004, the Associated Press reported that pharmaceutical companies would be required to add the warning to HRT labels about this risk, in addition to the increased risk of breast cancer, heart attacks and strokes, already included in the warnings. On July 11, 2005, a study was reported warning those at risk for heart disease that taking birth control pills doubles the risk of heart attack and stroke.

New York Cardiologist Nieca Goldberg says: "even young women who begin using oral contraceptives should be screened for heart disease."

Men are also at risk for dementia due to hormone imbalance, according to a report in the *Journal of the American Medical Association*, February 2005. The study measured postmortem brain testosterone levels, and found a correlation between low levels of testosterone and preceding dementia in men. The results of the study are limited due to the fact that a single hormone was measured, rather than hormone balance, and there was no record of drugs taken prior to death. Morphine has an immediate effect on hormone levels, and could have been a mediating factor in this study. Interpretation of such data becomes critical, as two million prescriptions were written for testosterone replacement therapy in 2001.

Dr. Elizabeth Vliet, whose women's health clinics in Tucson, Arizona and Ft. Worth, Texas, focus on hormone balance to treat chronic illness, advises women to pay special attention to changes in brain function. She says, "The brain is often the first organ to show the effects of subtle changes in either thyroid or ovarian hormone function because the brain is so exquisitely dependent upon normal balance for optimal function. When I talk with physicians about these issues, I emphasize that the overall 'pattern' is what helps determine the tests to do."

Dr. Vliet also comments throughout her book about the superior results she sees in her patients when they exchange their synthetic hormone replacement therapy for native human estradiol and natural progesterone, because "it fits, like a key in a lock, at the specific brain receptor sites which help to regulate memory and information processing."

Using Progesterone for Uterine Fibroid Tumors

Estrogen is the "food supply" that causes fibroid tumors to grow. What women need to know is that fibroid tumors NEVER turn into cancer, but shrink and go away with the onset of menopause. The reason is simple. The "food supply" or estrogen levels decline once you start menopause. The problem with fibroid tumors is that they can contribute to heavy bleeding and painful periods. Although it has not been proven, I believe that since progesterone opposes the action of estrogen, it is conceivable that regular progesterone use over time would in fact decrease the size of a fibroid tumor. This is an area of progesterone therapy I have wanted to study for quite some time, after clinically seeing women with fibroids substantially improve. I recommend using 20mg of progesterone daily or cyclically (day 14 – 28) or the second half of the cycle after ovulation for fibroid tumors.

Using Progesterone for Fibrocystic Breast Disease

Fibrocystic breast disease is another symptom of too much estrogen in the system and it seems to affect mainly women of childbearing years. Progesterone is an easy answer for treatment, because it opposes the action or blocks the action of estrogen at the cell. These women suffer from very tender or painful breast tissue that may or may not worsen at certain times in their menstrual cycle. The breast tissue is not only tender it also may feel lumpy to the touch. Many of these women feel what they think is a "mass" and end up with needle biopsy to find out that the mass is a cyst. The response to progesterone is pretty rapid and many women can tell a difference in 1-3 months. Using 20mg of progesterone daily or cyclically will usually alleviate the problem.

Menstrual Migraines

Some women experience migraine headaches that are cyclical in nature. Cyclical migraines are definitely hormone-related. They are usually due to excess estrogen and can be alleviated with the regular use of progesterone and 10-20mg of transdermal progesterone daily is usually sufficient to alleviate them. The progesterone can be used all month except when menstruating or it can be used in a cyclical fashion to more closely mimic what a normal cycle would do. To use it cyclically, use 10-20 mg on days 12-26 of your cycle.

Using Progesterone in Breast Cancer

There is considerable controversy on this topic, but after much research and inquiry I agree with a growing number of physicians that progesterone is breast protective. If you or a loved one has been diagnosed with breast cancer or is a breast cancer survivor, I strongly recommend that you read Dr. John Lee's and David Zava, PhD's book, *What Your Doctor May Not Tell You About Breast Cancer*. They point out much of the controversy in this area stems from the medical community's confusion between progestin and progesterone. Again, progestin is a synthetic, man-made version of progesterone. They are not the same hormone at all. Progestins are classified by the International Agency for Research on Cancer (IARC) as carcinogenic to humans. Progesterone is the hormone that all women make in their own bodies and for which there are receptors on every cell in our body whether it be a brain cell, a bone cell, a breast cell, etc!

It is so important that as a society and medical community, we stop confusing these two. Bioidentical progesterone and non-bioidentical progestin cannot be lumped together. When looking at the biochemical structure of progesterone, it more closely resembles testosterone than it does progestin! Yet how different progesterone is from testosterone! It has become clear to us that when a woman is diagnosed with an estrogen positive and progesterone positive breast cancer that the progesterone receptors are the body's natural attempt to ward off or get rid of that cancer! It has been shown that a woman with a progesterone deficiency has a 10-

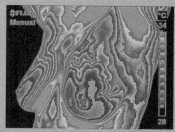

breastthermography.com

Thermography is a completely non-invasive breast health screening—no radiation, no compression, no pain. It uses a highly sensitive infrared camera to detect inflammation in the breast. Like a fingerprint, the "heat signature" of the breast is remarkably stable over time, and any change in that thermal fingerprint indicates that breast health problems are developing. Dr. Christine Horner, breast surgeon and spokesperson for the American Cancer Society says "it's an incredibly useful tool." In her book, she writes: "Research shows that, unlike mammograms, when thermography suspects something is wrong, it usually is. A study published in the American Journal of Radiology in January 2003 concluded that this technology could help prevent most unnecessary breast biopsies." For more information on the benefits of thermography visit: ***breastresearchawareness.com*** fold increased risk of all malignant neoplasms compared to a woman without a progesterone deficiency.

It is also critical that any woman concerned with reducing breast cancer risk understand the importance of adrenal gland function. If a woman has high cortisol levels at night (which may be seen with adrenal fatigue) she will not be able to make melatonin. She will likely also suffer from insomnia or is just not able to go to bed until well after midnight. She probably feels like she can't even get out of bed in the morning. The problem with this is that melatonin stimulates the production/activation of Natural Killer Cells (NKC). NKC are cancer scavengers within our body. A woman with compromised adrenal glands, who has a suppressed cortisol level all day long and a higher cortisol level at night is putting herself at risk for cancer. I am including a section on adrenal fatigue and thyroid disease because it is critical to overall health.

Adrenal Fatigue

Adrenal fatigue is a condition that can often interfere with hormone balance. Physicians have greatly underestimated the role of the adrenal glands. In medical school I was primarily taught that it either works or it doesn't; end of story. This is simply not the case and, as with many diseases, there is a progression of the disease. To categorize it as working or non-working is too simplistic. Similar to diabetes, there is a continuum from health to disease and variations of the disease. Some of the symptoms of adrenal fatigue are feeling tired in the morning, fatigue not relieved by sleep, increased effort to do daily tasks, craving salty foods, lethargy, decreased ability to handle stress and decreased sex drive. Additional symptoms can include depression, increased time to recover from illness, injury or trauma, feeling light-headed when you stand up quickly, less a sense of wellbeing, less enjoyment or happiness with life. Symptoms can worsen when meals are skipped, decreased tolerance, memory less accurate, fuzzy thinking and more!

Are you not awake until 10 in the morning, then need a ton of coffee or "energy" drinks, etc.? Are you only really awake after lunch? Do you have a mid-afternoon sinker? Are you at your best after 6 in the evening, but tired at 9 to 10, but resist sleeping? Do you get a burst of energy at 11-2 am - doing your "best" work in the wee hours? Then do you sleep late in the morning getting your best sleep at 7-9am? This is called ADRENAL FATIGUE. It is treatable and can also be found in children as well as adults. Drug moms can have adrenal fatigued infants.

James Wilson's book, Adrenal Fatigue–The 21st Century Stress Syndrome completely explains adrenal fatigue and offers treatments. If you have any of the above- mentioned symptoms, please get a copy of Dr. Wilson's book and educate yourself. Sometimes many symptoms of adrenal fatigue and female hormonal imbalance overlap. So it is essential to determine whether or not you may be suffering from adrenal fatigue to achieve optimal hormone balance, health and wellbeing.

Thyroid Disorders

It seems that the standard approach to diagnosing and treating thyroid disorders is a bit erroneous in traditional medicine too. Traditionally doctors are taught to measure a TSH (thyroid stimulating hormone) and, if it is within normal range, the person is declared normal. Yet many patients complain of low thyroid symptoms, go to the doctor's office to get checked for the disease only to be told they are "normal." The problem is they don't feel normal. The problem with this test is it does not check what is going on in the thyroid or in the tissues! TSH tells us that the brain is functioning, but what about the thyroid gland? Too many times people can even present with a goiter on their thyroid gland and are told they are "normal" because their TSH is fine.

One problem with this type of thinking is explained in the way lab test "normal" is created. Scientists create a range of what is normal for a population by testing a large group of people from all age ranges. Ninety-five percent of the population will have an average TSH between 0.4 and 4.5, for example. In general, the lower the TSH the higher the thyroid levels in the bloodstream. However, as we age our thyroid function often declines and people who have a deficient thyroid are also included in the measurement. So, as a result, the so-called "normal" can be off. I always strive for a TSH around 1.0, which is closer to the value seen in people with a youthful, fully functional thyroid gland. It is also critical to check a free T4 level, free T3 level, thyroid antibodies and sometimes a thyroid binding globulin.

These thyroid function markers can be checked with traditional blood work or through the blood spot method mentioned earlier. If the thyroid antibodies are elevated, even if your thyroid markers are otherwise normal, you may have early autoimmune thyroid disease. T4 is the precursor form of thyroid hormone. That is what is found in the prescription medication Synthroid®. It has four iodine molecules on it, thus T4. The body converts T4 to T3 by cleaving off one of the iodine molecules. Before thyroid hormone can be utilized by the peripheral tissues and perform its functions, it must be converted to T3. Some people have trouble converting free T4 to T3 and this can be the problem that is causing their symptoms. If a man or woman seeks to balance their hormones, he/she must make sure that the thyroid hormones are in balance and adrenal glands are functioning properly. Otherwise hormone balance can be forever elusive.

Problem Skin and Hormones

Skin "problems" are often the physical evidence of a heavy toxin load blocking or overwhelming other elimination points. We often look for a little dab of medicinal fix-it to paint on a blemish to quickly remedy an unsightly pimple, but pimples erupting on the skin may be toxins expressing through the skin and could signal something that may require more than topical skin treatments.

Skin problems let us know that hormones are likely out of balance, or that foods may be unmanageable by our body, and/or toxins are brimming to the top and spilling over onto the skin because the liver, the largest internal detoxifying system, is overloaded. Problem skin alerts us to malfunctions in the body, thereby signaling us to take remedial steps to avoid chronic problems with body systems.

Forty to fifty million people in the U.S. have acne. While acne is considered to plague only teenagers, many people over the age of 25 suffer from acne; 54 percent of women and 40 percent of men have some degree of acne, and children as young as 4 years old have been diagnosed. U.S. consumers spend $100 million on over-the-counter acne remedies per year to treat their symptoms. But what causes acne? Is it possible to "cure" acne if we treat the cause?

The answer is yes according to Dr. Loren Cordain. Acne, says Cordain, is a result of the combination of diet and hormones that affect the skin's life cycles. Certain popular foods can increase androgens (male hormones) in the blood, causing the body to produce more oil, or sebum. Overproduction of sebum in pores contributes to acne, causing bacteria to colonize, which raises the level of inflammation and infection. The immune system kicks in and produces pro-inflammatory hormones called cytokines, resulting in a papule, pustules, or nodule (bumps, spots, or zits). In essence, the body's entire delicate balance of hormones is thrown out of sync by a chain reaction linked to diet.

The food culprits that trigger this domino effect are not limited to a single food group. Diets heavy in carbohydrates contribute to the delay in cell death (apoptosis), because carbohydrates rapidly increase insulin levels in the body. Carbohydrates can also be high glycemic-load foods, which elevate androgens in the blood stream and, and as previously noted, create an overabundance of oil produced by the skin.

The Harvard School of Public Health demonstrated that milk, so common to the American diet, is associated with acne in a group of 47,355 women in the Nurse's Health Study. Hormones can be disrupted as the body breaks down the foods we don't necessarily need as adults, like milk, but it is also possible to consume strong growth hormones fed to cows from the milk that we drink. Milk also has the ability to impair zinc absorption, a necessary nutrient in the skin's arsenal of defenses. Dairy products also induce high levels of insulin, leading to the same sequence of events caused by carbohydrates, ultimately leading to acne.

In addition to carbohydrates, fats can cause a number of responses related to acne. Americans consume ten times more omega-6 (corn oil, canola oil, etc.) than omega-3 oils (10:1), found in foods like sardines, salmon, flax seeds and walnuts, while the ideal ratio of omega-6 to omega-3 is 2:1. This 10:1 ratio produces a constant pro-inflammation in many body tissues, resulting in an immune response to invading bacteria perpetuating the acne cycle.

Men, Progesterone & Testosterone

Like women, men make all three sex hormones: estrogen, progesterone and testosterone. Testosterone is the primary androgen that men need for optimal health, and progesterone is the precursor hormone men need to maintain healthy levels of testosterone. Men experience a natural decline in testosterone beginning as early as their mid-thirties, which can lead to an excess of estrogen. About half of men will begin experiencing symptoms of testosterone deficiency in their 50's. Symptoms of testosterone deficiency include decreased libido, mood disturbances, depression, fatigue, loss of muscle size and strength, osteoporosis, increased body fat, frequent urination and prostate enlargement, memory loss and sleep difficulty. Dr. Eugene Shippen author of the The Testosterone Syndrome says:

> *If I told you that one key substance in the body is more powerful than any other health factor, is more closely linked to risk of illness if and when deficiency occurs, is more misunderstood, more improperly used, and more tragically underused than any other, what would it be? Testosterone! I have studied it, prescribed it, and watched the responses of my patients-hundreds of them. I challenge anyone to find a more diversely positive*

Questions for Treatment:
Do you currently have or ever had any of the following symptoms?

Sex Function		
Decrease in spontaneous early morning erections.	YES	NO
Decrease libido or desire for sex.	YES	NO
Decrease in fullness of erections.	YES	NO
Decrease in volume of ejaculate or semen.	YES	NO
Decrease in strength of climax or force of muscular pulsations.	YES	NO
Difficulty in maintaining full erection.	YES	NO
Difficulty in starting erection-or no erection.	YES	NO
Mental Functions		
Spells of mental fatigue or inability to concentrate; feeling burned out.	YES	NO
Tiredness or sleepiness in the afternoon or early evening.	YES	NO
Decrease in mental sharpness, attention, wit.	YES	NO
Change in creativity or spontaneous new ideas.	YES	NO
Decrease in initiative or desire to start new projects.	YES	NO
Decreased interest in past hobbies or new work-related activities.	YES	NO
Decrease in competitiveness.	YES	NO
Change in memory function; increased forgetfulness.	YES	NO
Feelings of depression.	YES	NO
Musculoskeletal Condition		
"Sore-body syndrome"-aches, joint and muscle pain.	YES	NO
Decline in flexibility and mobility; increased stiffness.	YES	NO
Decrease in muscle size, tone, strength.	YES	NO
Decrease in physical stamina.	YES	NO
Decrease in athletic performance.	YES	NO
Back pain; neck pain.	YES	NO
Tendency to pull muscles or get leg cramps.	YES	NO
Development of osteoporosis or inflammatory arthritis.	YES	NO
Metabolic or Physical/Disease Problems		
Increase in total cholesterol or triglycerides.	YES	NO
Decrease in HDL cholesterol.	YES	NO
Rise in blood sugar level diabetes onset.	YES	NO
Rise in blood pressure/ diagnosis of hypertension.	YES	NO
Unexplained weight gain, particularly in the midsection; "beer belly".	YES	NO
Increased fat distribution in breast area or hips.	YES	NO
Development of chest pain, or diagnosis of heart disease or blockage of arteries.	YES	NO
Shortness of breath with activities; worsening of asthma or emphysema.	YES	NO
Lightheadedness, dizzy spells, ringing of the ears; new onset of headaches.	YES	NO
Poor circulation in legs, swelling of ankles, varicose veins or hemorrhoids.	YES	NO
Changes in visual acuity focus reading fine print.	YES	NO

Excerpts from "The Testosterone Syndrome: The Critical Factor for Energy, Health, and Sexuality "
by Eugene Shippen, MD
(Paperback - Jan. 25, 2001)

factor in men's health. When normally abundant, it is at the core of energy, stamina, and sexuality. When deficient, it is at the core of disease and early demise.

Dr. John Lee, who is best known for his research with women and bioidentical progesterone, also recommends progesterone for men:

It is well known that the estradiol level in 55-year old men, for example, is usually a bit higher than that of a 55-year old woman. The man, however, does not develop breasts because he has a higher testosterone level than women do. As men age, their estradiol levels gradually rise, whereas their progesterone and testosterone levels gradually fall. The hormone balance changes. These gradual changes lead to reduction in testosterone benefits and eventually to estrogen dominance. That is, his estradiol effects emerge since his testosterone level is not sufficient to block or balance them.

Prostate Cancer

Prostate cancer occurs, in part, because testosterone and progesterone levels fall with age and estrogen levels rise, leading to estrogen dominance in older men. Of the three estrogens, estradiol in particular is harmful to a man's prostate because it causes the prostate to enlarge and likely is one of the main causes of prostate cancer. Like women, men are often prescribed diuretics and other pharmaceuticals to address prostate enlargement and the resulting frequent urination, without getting to the root of the hormone imbalance. Progesterone is a precursor and regulator for the production of testosterone. Progesterone inhibits the conversion of testosterone to di-hydro-testosterone (DHT) just like the drug, Proscar® and Saw Palmetto. Only progesterone is a much more potent inhibitor of this detrimental conversion. Higher levels of DHT and lower levels of testosterone are associated with prostate enlargement (BPH), prostate cancer and balding. High DHT levels are found in the enlarged prostate, and in the hair follicles in primary male pattern baldness. Therefore, progesterone could benefit in all these conditions. Dr. Lee recommends 10 mg of bioidentical transdermal progesterone applied directly to the scrotum twice daily as helpful in balancing the ratio of testosterone to the increasing estrogen levels in a man's body as well as to maintain bone strength.

Similar mechanisms that cause breast cancer and uterine cancer in women cause prostate cancer in men. Prostate problems are the fastest-growing health concern in Westernized countries; and the rate of prostate cancer is increasing steadily. One man in six will be diagnosed with prostate cancer in his lifetime, and one in thirty-six will die from prostate cancer. It is the second leading cause of cancer death in men.

Causal factors are thought to include estrogen dominance (particularly from exposure to soy, dairy, hormone exposed meat and xenoestrogens in personal care products), testosterone deficiency, lack of sexual activity, zinc deficiency and insufficient nighttime sleep. A good night's sleep is so vital to health for many reasons, but as mentioned previously, there is a beneficial effect of melatonin on natural killer cells (NKC). NKC are immune cells that seek out and kill any precancerous cells in the body. NKC activity is stimulated by the hormone melatonin which is produced primarily while you are in a deep sleep. So not only should we get our beauty rest for looking our best, but also for good health.

There is much said today about "the environment", but most of us don't realize how close pollution is to us, nor do we understand the current and future implications for a petrochemical-based society, which represents most of the developed world. I have begun following news reports and conducting research on largely unseen hormone aspects of "pollution," a problem that applies to both men and women.

Vitamin D: An Essential Hormone for Reproductive Organ Health

Vitamin D, a hormone normally produced in the skin using energy from sunlight, has taken center stage in nutrition research, and for good reason. It is associated with improved health in all four of the top chronic illnesses in America, hypertension, diabetes, heart disease, and cancer. When evaluating research findings, it is important to have a large sample size, and to control every possible factor that could influence the outcome. These robust and controlled University studies have found significant health benefits associated with a high blood serum level of Vitamin D, and many recommend a supplement of 4,000 units per day, especially in the winter when sun exposure is limited. The following are a list of health factors affects by Vitamin D:

- **Type 1 Diabetes**

    According to a 2009 article in Britain's premier medical journal, *The Lancet*, Type I Diabetes in children younger than five could double by the year 2020. In his book, *Diabetes Rising*, Dan Hurley [who has lived with Type I Diabetes all his life] writes about the current theories that would explain the fastest growing disease in history—diabetes. He describes these factors as "fertilizers" affecting the genetic tendency to have diabetes, similar to how others have written about the Western diet "triggers" that change the health of one culture over another.

    First, children that grow faster, have more body stress, which can overwork the organs, and larger children have more diabetes. Vitamin D is also a factor. Countries nearer the equator have lower rates, and within the U.S., Minnesota rates of diabetes are much higher than Southern California. There is research pointing to exposure to germs and parasites that could build a resistance to diabetes. It is being studied with other autoimmune diseases in the UK such as multiple sclerosis and ulcerative colitis.

Type I Diabetes is an autoimmune disease, and cow's milk exposure may be a trigger in autoimmune diseases. Babies exposed to infant formula containing cow's milk in the first six months of life have a poorer developed immune system. One researcher interviewed by Hurley stated that using a hydrolyzed formula instead of cow's milk would likely cut the rate of infant diabetes by one fifth. Finally, Hurley found that pollution appears to have an influence on diabetes, but much more so in adult onset Type II diabetes.

- **Uterine Tumors**

  A study conducted by the National Institutes of Health found that women who had sufficient Vitamin D were 32 percent less likely to develop fibroid tumors in the uterus. These fibroids are the leading cause of hysterectomy in the United States. The study sample was 1,036 women ages 35-49. Those who reported spending more than one hour per day in the sun had an estimated reduction in tumors of 40 percent. [1]

- **Premenopausal Breast Cancer**

  A University of California study involving 1,200 healthy women found that women whose serum Vitamin D level was low during the three month period before diagnosis had approximately three times the risk of breast cancer as women in the highest Vitamin D group. The study was published in the journal, *Cancer Causes and Control*.

- **Bone and Muscle Health**

  A UK study conducted by researchers from Newcastle University found that Vitamin D is vital for combating poor bone health and muscle fatigue. The researchers concluded that Vitamin D enhances the activity of mitochondria in the cells, where energy metabolism occurs. Patients took oral Vitamin D for 10 to 12 weeks, and reduced the phosphocreatine recovery time in the muscle by 18 percent. Doctors reported that 60% of people living north of Manchester are Vitamin D deficient, and could boost energy levels by taking a Vitamin D supplement.[2]

---

1   Baird, D.D., et al. 2013. *Vitamin D and the risk of uterine fibroids.* Epidemiology; 24(3): 447-453. NIH/ National Institute of Environmental Health Sciences.

2   Newcastle University. *"Poor Bone Health, Muscle Fatigue Due to Vitamin D Deficiency Effectively Treated with Supplements."* Medical News Today, April 8, 2013.

- **Obesity in Children**

  Although a small sample study, the University of Missouri Columbia treated 35 pre-diabetic obese children and adolescents with Vitamin D. Dr. Peterson explained that obese individuals process Vitamin D about half as efficiently as normal-weight people. The vitamin gets stored in their fat tissues, which keeps it from being processed, so they need twice as much to maintain sufficient levels. The researchers found that Vitamin D supplements can help obese children control their blood-sugar levels, which can lower their risk for developing Type 2 diabetes, and help to overcome insulin resistance, which is associated with obesity. The study was published in the *American Journal of Clinical Nutrition*.

- **Complications of Pregnancy**

  Canadian researchers conducted a survey of 31 studies published between 1980 and 2012 reporting the effects of Vitamin D supplementation during pregnancy. They report that Vitamin D deficiency is linked to risk of infection, preeclampsia, gestational diabetes, fetal growth restriction, cesarean section, and low birth weight for newborns. An elevated level of Vitamin D during pregnancy was associated with the prevention of multiple sclerosis later in the mothers.[3]

- **Childhood Diseases**

  A British study recommended widespread Vitamin D supplements, warning that half of the UK's white population, and up to 90% of the multi-ethnic population are vitamin D deficient, resulting in higher incidence of diabetes, tuberculosis, multiple sclerosis, and rickets. The country's chief medical officer recommended that all pregnant and breastfeeding women, children ages 6 months to five years, and people ages 65 and over should take Vitamin D supplements. They recommended that health care professionals be trained in spotting signs of Vitamin D deficiency in children; aches and pains, poor growth, muscle weakness, and seizures.[4]

- **Lung Function and Pneumonia**

  The *Journal of Clinical Endocrinology & Metabolism* reports a study of 10,000 Korean adults, which found that the absorption of Vitamin D improves lung function. People with a history of tuberculosis of the lungs had significantly lower levels of serum Vitamin D.

---

3 Robyn Lucas, et al. *Vitamin D. sufficiency in Pregnancy.* BMJ 2013; 346. Cited in Medical News Today, March 27, 2013.

4 Royal College of Paediatrics and Child Health. *"Widespread Supplementation Needed to Halt Rise in Vitamin D Related Diseases in Children."* Medical News Today, December 17, 2012.

A study of 1,421 subjects in Eastern Finland demonstrated that low serum levels of Vitamin D are a risk factor for pneumonia. The risk was 2.5 times higher in subjects with the lowest vitamin D levels than in subjects with high vitamin D levels. Earlier research showed that Vitamin D deficiency weakens the immune system and increases the risk of mild respiratory infections.[5]

- **Hypertension**

  The American Heart Association journal, Hypertension, published a study showing that Vitamin D modestly reduced systolic blood pressure among 250 African American adults studied at seven major teaching hospitals.

- **Brain Function**

  The abnormal protein amyloid-beta is found in sticky plaques that clog up the space between brain cells in people with Alzheimer's. UCLA researchers found in a small pilot study that Vitamin D3 and omega 3 fatty acids help the immune system clear the brain of this abnormal protein. Their ground-breaking research was published in the Journal of Alzheimer's Disease in February, 2013.

- **Mortality**

  A robust study published in the European Heart Journal, May 2013, followed 5,409 older men in the UK for 13 years. 1,358 died from vascular and 1,857 from non-vascular causes. The researchers found that a double concentration of Vitamin D was associated with 20% lower vascular and 23% lower non-vascular mortality. A meta-analysis of other studies comparing the top and bottom quarter of Vitamin D concentration revealed a 21% lower vascular and 28% lower all-cause mortality.

Endocrine Disruptors & Pollution

There are thousands of studies that show the adverse hormonal effects of petrochemical pollutants which originate outside the body, but which find their way inside the body through drinking water, the air we breathe, and the lotions, creams and make-up we put on our skin. These pollutants disrupt the delicate endocrine system, which manages the glands that make brain hormones, reproductive hormones, adrenal hormones, as well as insulin and thyroid hormones. For simplified discussion here, these endocrine disrupters or EDs have an estrogen-like effect upon the body. Some or all hormone imbalance may be due to these environmental

---

5   University of Eastern Finland. *"Link between low vitamin D levels and pneumonia risk." Journal of Epidemiology and Community Health.* Cited in Medical News Today, May 2, 2013.

factors. The concern over these pollutants is the effect they have upon the reproductive organs of all living creatures. False estrogens are fat-soluble and non-biodegradable and easily pass through the skin to be stored in body fat. The more fat you have stored, the more likely you are to experience symptoms of estrogen dominance. There are some solutions to the problem so start by paying attention to the foods you eat. Animals are fattened up with hormones and eat grains grown with pesticides. These hormones and pesticides are stored in the animal's fat, so it's best to buy organic grass-fed meat, organic vegetables and drink filtered water.

- **Male Feminization**

  In 2003, a news story reported that 30 percent of male fish in the Potomac River were producing eggs, quite obviously a female fish function. In 2010, the follow up report appeared on the same fish study. The research then showed that nearly 80 percent of the male fish in the Potomac River were producing eggs! The researchers concluded in 2003 and again in 2010, that the male fish are being "feminized" due to exposure to chemicals that include synthetic hormones (birth control and hormone replacement therapy – excreted into the water system and then into lakes and streams) as well as the run off into waterways from feed lots where livestock excrete growth hormones, and also the use of industrial and chemicals components found in plastics, fertilizers, insecticides, fungicides etc., which are also making their way into the streams and rivers from which the public water supply is drawn.

  The Potomac Conservancy as well as the U.S. Geological Survey followed this and other similar studies. In 2010, the U.S. Geological Survey found "intersex" fish in one third of 111 sites tested around the country as powerful chemicals make their way into our waterways and greatly alter the natural function of life; and, uniformly, the finger of blame seems to unfailingly point to birth control pills as the primary culprit.

- **Submerged in EDCs - The Role of Environmental Toxins**

  Toxic chemicals have increased at an exponential rate over the past 50 years, with an average of 10 new chemicals introduced each day. The Environmental Protection Agency estimates that 87,000 chemicals are in widespread use and 2.2 million pounds of pesticides are sprayed on crops each year. We also know 85 billion pounds of plastic products are produced annually. The average American home contains 3-10 gallons of hazardous materials and 85% of the chemicals that are registered have never been tested for impact on the human body. Many of these chemicals are used on and in our bodies as personal care products. There are a number of studies pointing to environmental toxins as a causal factor in behavioral and developmental issues.

Further studies found these same substances present in human milk, placenta and umbilical cord blood, and in the blood and body fat of newborns. Phthalates, found in hundreds of products including soft vinyl plastic toys, shampoos, hair spray, nail polish, perfumes, new cars, pharmaceuticals and deodorants are known hormone disrupters that can cause sperm and genital problems in males and they were found in 75% of human urines tested.

In short, this is the environmental dilemma today: too much estrogen and other growth hormones make it very difficult to balance one's hormones, but there is more to the story. Males in many, if not all species of animal life could in effect be chemically neutered. What does this phenomenon called by a Canadian documentary "The Disappearing Male," [free viewing available online] mean for our own species 100 years from now, if something isn't done to clean up our act?

In the modern world we are literally submerged in EDCs, or Endocrine Disrupting Compounds. These are compounds that have the ability to disrupt the endocrine system, or the hormonal system. Over 80,000 EDCs are in use in commerce, farming and industry. According to the National Institute of Environmental Health Sciences (NIEHS):

> "Pharmaceuticals, fabric treatments, pesticides, fertilizers and other chemicals can disrupt the endocrine systems and can be found in water…. Exposure to environmental chemicals, including EDC's in the environment may play an important role in the etiology of diseases….along with nutrition, infection and stress."

So far filtering out EDCs from our public water system is difficult, if not impossible. Water treatment systems in the U.S. were designed to eliminate harmful bacteria, not designed to filter out an array of pharmaceuticals, hormones and other chemicals. Consequently, here is a short list of some of the household products found in our environment, and more troubling specifically in our water:

- Anti-inflammatories/analgesics like ibuprofen, naproxen, aspirin
- Seizure medications
- Psychiatric medications and antidepressants
- Cholesterol medications
- Synthetic hormones including 17 alphaethinyl estradiol, 17 beta estradiol, and estrone
- Pesticides, organophosphates, carbamates, pyrethroids, organochlorine

- Blood pressure medicines like metoprolol and atenolol
- Antibiotics and antimicrobials including triclosan, sulphonamides, tetracycline
- Diuretics
- Personal care products that include insect repellants, preservatives, soaps, sunscreens, fragrances, cosmetics, toothpaste

To point out the importance of using pure and safe personal care products, look at a study in Massachusetts involving high school girls, who used cosmetics. Researchers drew and tested the teenage girls' blood and urine to assess the known levels of toxic chemicals present in the cosmetics.

Not surprising, there were alarmingly high levels of toxic but commonly used cosmetic chemicals. EDC's were found in the girl's blood and urine. The researchers stated many of these young women would go on to experience adverse health effects from an ongoing exposure to these chemicals and there would also be those who would struggle with hormonal imbalances and some would even go on to experience infertility. Like in the egg-producing "intersex" fish, EDCs impact the reproductive systems of young girls as well as their entire endocrine system causing problems like polycystic ovarian syndrome, insulin resistant diabetes, obesity, etc. More studies are needed to assess the impact of environmental toxin exposure on male infertility and testosterone imbalance, as well as the troubling increase in prostate dysfunction and cancer.

- **EDCs: An Explanation for Obesity Epidemic**

  Many of the EDC's are now considered "Obesogens," or an EDC that a child, for example, is exposed to in childhood that causes the child to become obese as an adult. This is seen with DES (Diethylstilbesterol) exposure. According to Newbold, et al, mice given DES for just 5 days at birth resulted in increased weight in female mice beginning at puberty. This is with absolutely no change in the food intake or exercise of these mice! Photos of their research show a massively obese mouse compared to its sibling not receiving DES for 5 days at birth. There are many chemicals that are now categorized as "obesogens." The obesogen's trigger is a short exposure during early development and leading to obesity later in life.

  Without getting too scientific here, what we're talking about is "Epigenetics," the study of "chemical" modifications of DNA and chromatin, which are heritable and affect genome function (transcription, replication, recombination), but do not affect the DNA backbone. What does that mean? It means simply that some chemicals to which we are exposed have the ability to modify our DNA and are able to be passed on to future generations.

Hormones and Fertility

Bioidentical progesterone can be used for female infertility, when the issue is anovulation or no ovulation. Progesterone is a widely accepted treatment for anovulation among fertility specialists. Generally, if a woman is not ovulating, it is because she has low progesterone levels. She may or may not have a period.

It is best to start out by using 20-40mg of USP Progesterone daily for 90 days, if you are not having a period. After the 90 days, stop using the progesterone and wait for a period. Once your period starts, begin using the progesterone on day 12 (of an average 28-day cycle) (at ovulation) through the start of your menstrual cycle. While most women do not have a 28-day cycle, I continue to use the 28-day cycle as a model in this book. The following guidelines are based on the average 28-day cycle and, again, may need adjusting for your particular cycle length.

For women not ovulating, but who are having a period, use 20-30mg of USP Progesterone on day 12 through the start of your period. The reason I recommend using the progesterone through the start of your period is that, if you are pregnant, we don't want to decrease the progesterone level. Some pregnant women with low progesterone levels, as many as 70 percent, suffer from frequent first trimester miscarriages. When an egg is fertilized just after ovulation it is the remnant that the egg leaves behind in the ovary that produces progesterone for the entire first trimester. During the second and third trimester the placenta takes over and produces large quantities of progesterone. Once you start your period you can stop using the progesterone and begin again at day 12 of the cycle. It is important to keep progesterone levels constant through the start of your period. If you do not start your period, take a pregnancy test and, if it is positive, continue using the progesterone. If you have had a first trimester miscarriage in the past, it is best to increase supplementation of progesterone, discussed in the next section.

Fertility is a measure of a person's overall health, and many dietary and chemical exposure issues affect both men's and women's ability to conceive. Only about half of infertile couples are able to identify a root cause, probably because so many dietary and environmental factors are working together to support fertility.

According to the U.S. Census Bureau, infertility among women in their 40's has increased 89 percent over the past three decades. Studies have suggested that birth control can produce irreversible infertility. Chlamydia infection is also a factor in both men and women, and the fact that it is often asymptomatic in men means that the damage it does to approximately one third of normal spermatozoa likewise goes undetected, unlike females who suffer from pelvic inflammatory disease and debilitating pain. Studies suggest that infertility is linked to hormone imbalance, the multitude of new varieties of sexually transmitted disease, chemical water treatment, food additives, and injury from birth control, both chemical and mechanical. While no one can definitively announce the cause, it is abundantly clear that the problem is immense, and the increase is steadily moving upward. It is cause for alarm and intervention, even if all the evidence is not in yet.

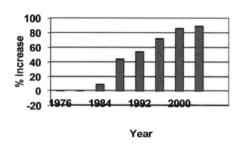

Percent Increase in Infertility 1976-2000

Balanced hormones are essential to conception, and numerous studies have demonstrated that women need progesterone to support the luteal phase when a fertilized egg is implanted in the uterus. Progesterone prepares the lining of the uterus for implantation and prepares the environment for a fertilized egg to grow. Low progesterone is associated with early miscarriage. Pregnant women have 200 times the level of progesterone as non-pregnant women. In addition, using bioidentical progesterone improves adrenal function, balances adrenal hormones including DHEA, and improves thyroid function, all necessary for conception. Progesterone balances the effects of estrogen and signals the release of insulin. In 1981, a study from Johns Hopkins concluded that women low in natural progesterone have an 80% higher risk of developing breast cancer and a ten-fold increase in other malignant cancers.

Also, excess testosterone in women can cause infertility. Balancing other hormones may be all that is necessary to bring the testosterone level down. Small studies have suggested that Saw Palmetto and other Chinese herbal preparations may be beneficial in lowering testosterone.

Over 1,000 chemicals have been identified that have an effect on fertility in animals. Plastics production, welding, tobacco, and lead exposure have been shown to affect men by lowering sperm count, causing abnormally shaped sperm, and decreasing motility. Studies are ongoing to show the effect of electromagnetic radiation on sperm vitality. Cell phones are negatively associated with sperm health due to radiation exposure.   Glutathione, which Dr. Hyman refers to as "the mother of all antioxidants" has been shown to increase sperm motility. The following is a short list of the most common hormone disruptors in our environment:

- Solvents & adhesives (paint, nail polish, household cleaners)
- Plastics
- Non-organic meats (they are given hormones to fatten up or to grow quicker)
- Pesticides, herbicides, fungicides
- Emulsifiers in soap and cosmetics
- Petrochemicals from industrial waste
- Hormonal birth control (pill, shot, ring, implant)

Men and Women- What to Avoid While Maximizing Fertility

Men	Women
Toxins	Toxins
Metal exposure	Antibiotics
Stress	Antidepressants
Alcohol	Aspirin and ibuprofen(esp. at mid-cycle)
Smoking	Chemical Birth control
Cell phone use	Stress
	Smoking
	Xenoestrogens
	Mercury
	Alcohol
	Caffeine in excess of 300 mg. / day

Suggested Supplements to Improve Fertility and Balance Hormones

Men	Women
Bioidentical progesterone	Bioidentical progesterone
Zinc (60 mg. daily	B vitamins (B2, B6, B12, folic acid)
Selenium	Vitamin C
Glutathione	Iron
Vitamin C (1000 mg. daily)	Prenatal vitamins for 6 mo. Prior to conception
Vitamin E (400 mg. daily)	
CoQ10 (100 mg. daily)	
Arginine (3,000 mg. daily)	
Carnitine (3,000 mg. daily)	
Ginseng (200 mg. daily)	

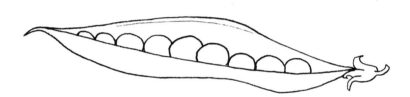

PCOS & Pregnancy
By D'Etta Thomas

At the age of 26, I was diagnosed with Polycystic Ovarian Syndrome. It didn't seem like a big deal then because I wasn't yet interested in starting a family. My doctor assured me I needed to go on a "low-estrogen" birth control pill to regulate my monthly cycles. She said to let her know when my husband and I wanted to get pregnant, because she had the pills I would need to make that happen, which went in one ear and out the other.

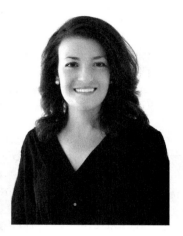

Fast forward to 2010, I went off of birth control. I thought I'm healthy, I'm thin, I'm active, and I don't suffer from any condition, so I'm sure I'll be able to get pregnant on my own." Wrong. But I convinced myself it was no big deal that I didn't understand when I was or wasn't ovulating. I would hear my friends say 'I always ovulate on day blah to day blah of my cycle…' and I would always nod as if I was following what they were saying, but truthfully I had no clue!? How did they know? What am I missing?

I went online and ordered a book my friend recommended called "Taking Charge of Your Fertility" by Toni Weschler, MPH. A light bulb snapped on after reading it – I don't ovulate! Why? Something really is wrong with me! Then my best friend, Cindy Peterson, told me about bioidentical progesterone, molecularly like your body makes. It sounded good, but I wanted to ask my doctor. So back to the doctor I went. I told her that I took myself off of my birth control and I hadn't gotten pregnant. In fact, I hadn't even had a period since going off of the birth control!

My doctor prescribed a progesterone pill (progestin – not bioidentical like your body makes) and said "take this pill if you haven't had a period after 3 months. I don't want you going any longer than 3 months without having a cycle." I explained that I wanted to try a natural bioidentical progesterone. She shot me down saying, don't bother, it won't work and tells me that since a typical PCOS patient is overweight, sometimes obese, she can always tell them to lose weight and they'll get pregnant.

However in my case, I was a perfect weight and had no room to lose. She explained in my situation, the only assistance she could give me (without sending me to an IVF Clinic) would be to try a prescription drug called Metformin for several weeks and then to add in a prescription fertility pill (that was not FDA approved yet, yikes.)

I was hesitant about all of it. I walked out of that appointment with 3 prescriptions to fill! Sheesh. I also had my husband telling me to "stop trying to be the medical marvel and just take the pills!" Several times I did start on the progesterone pills and I did produce a period, yet I was still unable to ovulate during those cycles. I also took Metformin for almost 2 weeks but felt TERRIBLE. So I quit taking them.

With the prescriptions not working and me not ovulating, I now I had to understand the "WHY"? So I started to research myself. I found that most everyone with PCOS was also taking Metformin to regulate their blood sugar which helps start ovulation again. I couldn't understand why I would need a pill that is typically prescribed for a patient with diabetes; I didn't have diabetes. My blood work looked great! No signs of anything else. So my next question that I was going to find the answer to was 'how can I balance my blood sugars naturally?' Anything that I wanted to do naturally I knew would have to be found all on my own. Again, as my husband likes to say, I wanted to be a "medical marvel" and get pregnant naturally (pharmaceutical drug free).

So after long nights on my computer, I found something. And it was BIG. Huge! It was a simple pill called Inositol. Now I'm no doctor, but in the research I did, I was amazed that a natural substance could help increase progesterone, lower testosterone & help improve insulin sensitivity and much more! Sounded liked a natural alternative to Metformin to me! Sign me up!! I literally ran out & bought a bottle the very next day!

My new regimen was a natural alternative to the progesterone pill, bioidentical transdermal progesterone cream and the natural alternative to Metformin was Inositol. I also learned the absolute and critical importance of staying away from sugars/carbs and sticking to a low-glycemic diet. In fact, I ordered 3 cookbooks to help me stick to a low-glycemic diet. If these 3 alternatives truly worked, then I would have no need for a fertility pill.

The last thing I did was print off a fertility calendar. I wanted to document everything I was doing…when I started the bioidentical progesterone cream, when I started my vitamins & Inositol and what my basal temperature was every day. I figured I'd be doing this "documenting" for a couple of months before my body adjusted and absorbed all the necessary components to begin ovulation. Boy was I wrong. I started all my "medical marvel" treatments and on December 1st 2011, I had a positive pregnancy test mid-month of January 2012. The first thing my husband said when I

ran in the room with a stick full of pee to show him we're pregnant was, "how did we do that?" I said, "well…I'm a medical marvel!"

It's amazing what a little (or a lot) of self-education can do! I always tell my friends to be their own "doctor." Never take "no" as an answer & always look for a natural alternative! I'm eternally grateful to my best friend who gave me my free baby-in-a-bottle, bioidentical progesterone. I'm also grateful to the other pioneer women who posted their struggles & 'findings' online that benefited me so greatly. I, in turn, would like to share my own story so that I can help someone else. By the way, we were blessed with a healthy 8lb. baby on October 1st, 2012.

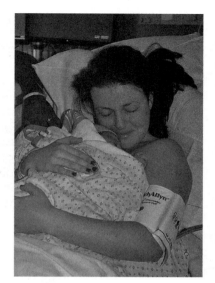

Education and Action

What should our response be to all of this?
In medicine it might simply mean changing our focus from curing a disease to prevention and intervention strategies to reduce disease incidence. In law it might mean changing the way industrial chemicals are now regulated. It might mean tighter regulatory control over the pharmaceutical industry. Currently of the 80,000 chemicals used in commerce, only 200 have been tested. U.S. government safety agencies generally consider chemicals "innocent until proven guilty". That means a potentially harmful chemical could be in the market for 10 or more years before it is discovered to be a problem.

To the average American it is a wakeup call to be proactive and educated on health care/medication decisions. We must take the bull by the horns, so to speak. It is our responsibility to control what chemicals our families are exposed to in our foods, homes and environment. This means finding and buying good local produce, organic foods, avoiding household chemicals that are harmful, knowing where our meat comes from and how it is produced, filtering our own water, partnering with a personal care company that you know and can trust to use safe ingredients and to be transparent with ingredient policies and green commitments. It means educating oneself and taking action because your future, our future depends upon it.

Chapter 2 Recommendations:

- Use bioidentical USP Progesterone applied to the skin
- 10 mg daily for men for prostate health
- 20 mg. daily days 12-28 for menstruating women, all but five days of the calendar month for menopausal women
- Supplement with Vitamin D3, 4000 units daily, and a multivitamin and mineral supplement
- Test your hormone levels using saliva (ZRT Labs)
- Avoid chemical birth control
- Drink filtered water and avoid petrochemicals in skin care and cleaning products
- Avoid pesticides and chemical fertilizers
- Take the Braverman Test and follow supplement recommendations, if needed. The test is available online and can point to neurological issues.
- Thermography for breast cancer screening
- Balance hormones and check for food sensitivies before resorting to birth control as acne treatment
- To meet the environmental toxicity challenge to your body use a mild detox periodically to support the liver and cleanse the blood.
- Detox before trying to conceive.

Chapter 3
Gut Health to Restore Metabolism, Immunity and Wellbeing

There is a new and exciting focus on gut research that confirms the correlation between our health and the optimal function of the gut. This chapter is a compendium of research findings that have been reported in the last couple of years, and many more studies are in progress to sort out the importance of gut bacteria, the communication between the gut and brain, the immune system's dependence upon the gut, and more.

Mal-absorption may be a root cause of many new and confusing digestive maladies from Irritable Bowel Syndrome, Leaky Gut, to life threatening Celiac Disease and Crohn's Disease. Who had ever heard of the stunning myriad of food allergies and digestive issues in the young and old alike even a decade ago?

Gut maladies disrupt the body's ability to absorb nutrients properly and thereby maintain optimal nutritional support of the body. Further the incidence of inflammatory bowel disease and food allergies has increased 50 percent since the 1990's. Incidence of eczema and skin allergies have risen 69 percent, and now affects one in eight children.

When writing about cracking a code on disease and aging, surprisingly a most important system is indeed the gut. A renewed appreciation for gut health is on the rise after decades of misunderstanding. Michael Pollan in his book, *Cooked*, points out that since the work of microbiologist Louis Pasteur, antibiotics have been highly prized, but the devastating effect to the gut by antibiotics is ignored. We gained an unhealthy fear of molds, bacteria, trichinosis, botulism and countless other germs lurking in our foods and environments, when most of which are helpful and necessary to gut health and overall health and wellbeing. There are other challenges today besides antibiotics as we begin to explore restoring health and wellbeing through better guts.

Why is Gut Health Vital?

Most mid-life Westerners can only imagine feeling great and having plenty of energy throughout the day, having a clear mind, able to remember details, analyze information, having a noticeably keen sense of logic, being pain free and limber, no matter what your age, free of allergies and seldom, if ever, plagued by colds and flu, having clear and radiant skin, while also possessing a strong sense of wellbeing and not subject to roller coaster emotions that distract and decrease productivity. Could the forgoing description be the result of the condition of the ten trillion bacteria in your gut? The scientific research of the past two years answers that question with an emphatic "yes!"

Who knew the gut is so vital to the optimal function of all body systems? Who knew the gut was in large part the body's immune system, or that the gut does indeed play a significant role in autoimmune disease as well as depression and anxiety?

Today there are more and more people ready to look again, as Pollan says, at "the microcosmos" for its role in our overall health and wellbeing. Some who ferment foods, a great source of microbes for gut health, contend that human beings are really ambulatory devices for microbes, yet we have declared war on 99 percent of beneficial gut-protective bacteria with overuse of antibiotics, hand sanitizers, routine sterilization of food, etc. Pollan reports that "for the first time in history, it has become important to consciously replenish our microflora" to protect our health.

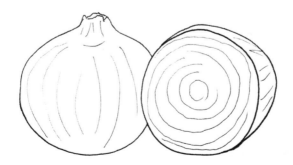

The Causes of Poor Gut Health

The Western Diet

Much is written about the "Standard American Diet" or the SAD and there are also a number of documentaries on the dangers of the SAD now popularly available via online services like Netflix and Hulu. The SAD diet is a pro-inflammatory diet that causes the body to have extremely high levels of inflammation as well as oxidative stress. It is now known that inflammation, oxidative stress and autoimmune disease play a significant role in hypertension, coronary artery disease, metabolic syndrome, thyroid disorders, arthritis, cancers, and so much more.

The SAD diet – what we eat - plays a significant role also in gut health. Dr. Emeran Mayer, professor at UCLA School of Medicine, led a study to examine the effect of ingesting probiotics on brain function. He reported, "There are studies showing that what we eat can alter the composition and products of the gut flora—in particular - people eating high-vegetable, fiber-based diets have a different composition of microbiota, or gut environment, than people who eat the more typical Western diet usually higher in fat and carbohydrates. Now we know that these foods have an effect not only on metabolism, but also on brain function."

Wheat

Today's wheat is altered and those changes to wheat affect gut health. Dr. William Davis, preventive cardiologist in Milwaukee, Wisconsin and author of *Wheat Belly*, views the changes to wheat as disastrous to human health. Over the past 50 years, Davis explains that wheat strains were altered to make the wheat resistant to environmental stress such as drought, as well as pathogens and fungi, with most genetic changes selected to increase yield per acre. Much of the current world supply of wheat is descended from strains developed in 1943 by Dr. Norman Borlaug who received the Nobel Prize for his high yield dwarf wheat. Borlaug's mission was to solve world hunger, a laudable goal, and he was very successful at increasing yield. Through his efforts China's wheat crop increased eight fold from 1961 to 1999. However, the "amber waves of grain" we sing of in "America" are no longer growing four feet high. Today's dwarf wheat now comprises 99 percent of all wheat grown worldwide.

Analyses of proteins expressed by this wheat hybrid compared to its two parent strains have demonstrated that five percent of its proteins are unique, found in neither parent strain. Referring to Borlaug's original research published in the Journal of Theoretical and Applied Genetics, Dr. Davis points out that modern strains of wheat produce a higher quantity of genes for gluten proteins that today are associated with celiac disease. The problem lies with wheat gluten in particular. It undergoes structural change with each hybridization, and because wheat has undergone tens of thousands of hybridizations, it can no longer grow in the wild and it requires commercial nitrate fertilizers and pesticides. As scientists insert or remove single genes to breed for disease resistance, pesticide resistance, cold or drought tolerance, and any variety of genetic characteristics, no one has studied what effect these changes have on overall human health both now and in the future.

The good news for 3rd world hunger is wheat's increased glycemic index provides robust levels of energy, but that is also problematic for the well-fed 1st World. The extent to which a food increases blood sugar relative to glucose (glycemic index 100) determines that food's glycemic index. Today's whole wheat bread has a glycemic index of 72, which means it increases blood sugar more than table sugar, which has a glycemic index of 59. Dr. Davis points out, "Aside from some extra fiber, eating two slices of whole wheat bread is really little different, and often worse, than drinking a can of sugar sweetened soda or eating a sugary candy bar." (*Wheat Belly*, p. 33).

As was pointed out in the Introduction, Americans are generally overweight. Dr. Davis says "wheat belly" is a phenomenon to be observed everywhere, and is rather simply explained. Wheat products elevate blood sugars more than virtually any other carbohydrate. Wheat's conversion to glucose is unavoidably accompanied by rising levels of insulin, which allows entry of glucose into cells, which convert the glucose to fat. The higher the blood glucose, the greater the insulin level and the more fat deposited, particularly abdominal fat. It is a damaging cycle.

It is critical to get fuel food from carbohydrates that do not cause a sudden spike in blood sugar and overload the pancreas. The fad "no carbohydrate" diets of the past decade do not line up with the body's need for fuel. That fuel is a simple six chain organic carbon, and the body makes it from virtually all foods we eat. Complex as well as simple carbs are decomposed in the process of metabolism until the end product, glucose, can be used at the cellular level for energy.

Sugar, the majority of which is produced from GMO sugar beets, is a simple carbohydrate that is broken down into glucose extremely quickly, causing an overload on the pancreas, which must produce the counteracting insulin to keep the body in balance. When too much glucose is present, the body must convert it to glycogen and store it--there is a limit to how much glucose, and how quickly glucose, is processed by the body. Both sugar and wheat are an exceptionally terrible way to feed the body glucose, because they immediately overload the system. Complex carbohydrates, such as vegetables and fruits are metabolized into glucose at the pace the body was designed to handle.

An alarming study reported in September 2013 in *The Wall Street Journal* describes the long-term effects of overloading the body's systems for handling glucose. Fatty liver disease that was once characteristic of adult alcoholics is now found in one in ten children whose obesity testifies to the chronic overload of dense artificial high glycemic foods. About 20% of people with fatty liver disease will progress to cirrhosis of the liver, which requires a liver transplant to sustain life. According to Dr. Vos, the lead researcher in the 2013 study, data from a national health study for elevated liver enzymes indicates the percentage of children in the sample suspected of having the disease grew to 10.7% between 2007 and 2010, from about 4% between 1988 and 1994. The problem appears to be escalating at an alarming rate. Research is needed to address the 2005 introduction of genetically modified sugar in processed foods, and the overall obesity epidemic in American children.

So what happens when the average American takes in 200 times as much sugar as the body can process? First of all, most sugar in the U.S. is produced from genetically modified sugar beets which have been doused with RoundUp. The body reads the altered DNA as a foreign substance, and has to filter and clean out the toxic glyphosate from the Roundup, a heavy burden on the liver and kidneys. Then the sugar turns quickly to glucose, spiking the blood glucose level, and the pancreas kicks in with insulin trying to keep up with the assault. This creates feelings of sluggishness--all energy being focused on digestion and management of the toxic load. Yes, the body runs on glucose, but it is designed to get that glucose from real food--not glyphosate saturated genetically modified sugar beets and high gluten high allergy wheat! This is an important distinction!

Livestrong.com reports that carbohydrates are a macronutrient that your body needs in high doses on a daily basis for proper functioning. When you eat complex carbohydrates, they get converted to

A six-month study reported in the Journal of Organic Systems (Vol. 8, No. 1, 2013) found that inflammation of the digestive tract is linked to genetically engineered corn and soy (GE). Researchers fed 84 pigs GE soy and corn, and 84 pigs non-GE feed for a period of 22.7 weeks, which is the lifespan of a commercial pig. According to the U.S. Dept. of Agriculture, 94% of soy grown in the U.S. is genetically engineered. When the pigs were slaughtered, researchers found that male GE-fed pigs were 4 times more likely to have stomach inflammation, and females were 2.2 times more likely to have stomach inflammation compared to the non-GE fed pigs. In addition, the female pigs had a 25% heavier uterus than non-GE fed females, which could be an indicator of hyperplasia, endometriosis, or cancer. Humans have a similar GI tract to pigs.

glycogen and either used immediately for energy, providing a steady dose of blood glucose, or they are stored in the muscles and liver for energy at a later time. Simple carbs, by contrast, cause a spike in blood sugar that quickly dissipates, leaving a person feeling hungry and fatigued.

Protein satisfies hunger, so a good balance of protein and complex carbohydrates are needed. For sustained energy, eat foods rich in complex carbs. There are a number of sources for getting complex carbs into our diet; quinoa, legumes, fruits, vegetables and whole grains, but wheat should be avoided. In America wheat today is like corn and soy—now completely different in its genetic structure compared to twenty years ago. So the bread and corn chips we get in restaurants and at the grocery, and the soy additives in many processed foods challenge our digestive systems as well as our protective cleansing organs, and likely make us gain weight.

What to do? Avoid wheat and the four main GMO's—corn, soy, sugar, and oil. Dr. William Davis reports that his patients who went on a wheat-free diet for three months reported that acid reflux disappeared and the cyclic cramping and diarrhea of irritable bowel syndrome were gone, energy improved, sleep was deeper, and rashes disappeared which had been present for many years. Also rheumatoid arthritis pain improved or disappeared, and asthma symptoms improved or resolved. Athletes reported better performance.

Antibiotics

Doctors prescribe antibiotics routinely and they are considered a huge boon to humankind. However, a study published in the journal *Gut* describes permanent changes in gut flora after taking antibiotics as gut bacteria diminishes even during treatment.

After antibiotics, when restoring gut flora, the bacteria have a lower capacity to produce proteins, and have deficiencies in their function, including the absorption of iron, digesting certain foods, and producing essential molecules. Researchers suggest there could be far reaching results - an interruption in the gut bacteria responsible for the interconnection between the liver and colon and the production of bile acids, hormones, and cholesterol derivatives.

A Swedish study led by Dr. Cecilia Jernberg found that short courses of antibiotics can leave behind normal gut bacteria with antibiotic resistant genes for as long as two years after the end of treatment and concludes that the side effects of antibiotic therapy are greater and far more severe than previously thought and that includes anyone who eats nonorganic meat exposed to frequent antibiotics. Unless specifically labeled otherwise, beef, chicken, turkey and farm raised fish are regularly fed antibiotics. In fact, eighty percent of all antibiotics consumed in the U.S. are by food animals. The FDA has set the following guidelines:

Authority: Sec. 512 of the Federal Food, Drug, and Cosmetic Act (21 U.S.C. 360b). Sec. 20.813

> *Enrofloxacin oral solution.*
>
> *(d) Conditions of use. It is used in drinking water as follows: (1) Chickens and turkeys--(i) Amount. 25 to50 parts per million of enrofloxacin in drinking water. (ii) Indications. Chickens: Control of mortality associated with Escherichia coli susceptible to enrofloxacin. Turkeys: Control of mortality associated with E. coli and Pasteurella multocida (fowl cholera) susceptible to enrofloxacin. (iii) Limitations. Do not use in laying hens producing eggs for human consumption. Administer medicated water continuously as sole source of drinking water for 3 to 7 days. Prepare fresh stock solution daily. Treated animals must not be slaughtered for food within 2 days of the last treatment. Individuals with a history of hypersensitivity to quinolones should avoid exposure to this product. Quinolones are especially dangerous to humans because their side effects are often disabling and permanent.*

Cipro and Levaquin are the most commonly prescribed quinolones. They are neurotoxic, causing frequent peripheral and central nervous system difficulties. Joint pain, especially in the hips, elbows, wrists, and ankles is common. The pain is often severe, and can last for months or years. This drug will deteriorate the cartilage all over the body, causing arthritic symptoms. It is not recommended for anyone who has symptoms of an autoimmune disorder such as Celiac, Crohns, lupus, or multiple sclerosis. It can also cause damage to the eyes. Its side effects are more severe than other antibiotics, because in addition to damaging the gut flora, it can cross the blood brain barrier. Originally intended for the treatment of Anthrax, it is now used for minor infections such as urinary tract and sinus infections. Adverse event reporting in Italy by

Professor Martin Blaser from New York University's (NYU) Langone Medical Center has been studying the long-term effects of antibiotics on gut flora. He writes:

"Early evidence from my lab and others hints that, sometimes, our friendly flora never fully recover. These long-term changes to the beneficial bacteria within people's bodies may even increase our susceptibility to infections and disease. Overuse of antibiotics could be fueling the dramatic increase in conditions such as obesity, type 1 diabetes, inflammatory bowel disease, allergies and asthma, which have more than doubled in many populations."

doctors showed fluoroquinolones among the top three prescribed drugs causing adverse neurological and psychiatric effects. Of the top ten drugs reported for side effects to the FDA in 2011, three were antibiotics—Levaquin, Cipro, and Bactrim.

Candidiasis

Antibiotic overuse has resulted in chronic and debilitating illnesses. One such condition, systemic candidiasis, or yeast overgrowth, occurs when the gut flora are damaged or destroyed by antibiotics and can no longer keep the body's healthy bacteria in balance. It was unknown until the introduction of antibiotics, birth control pills, HRT, and drugs used for IBS and other digestive disorders.

There is a gut balance between candida in the gut, bifidobacteria, and acidophilus. When gut bacteria are damaged, the candida multiplies out of control, and can break down the gut lining. In the blood stream, it can promote food allergy and fungal infection, as well as symptoms of fatigue, respiratory and digestive disorders, and autoimmune responses such as Addison's disease.

Dr. Amy Myers on www.MindBodyGreen.com reports that leaky gut can also result from the overgrowth of Candida caused by antibiotic use, which disrupts the balance between good and bad bacteria in the gut.

Candida is a fungus, which is a form of yeast. A very small amount of candida lives in your mouth and intestines and its job is to aid with digestion and nutrient absorption but, when overproduced, it breaks down the wall of the intestine and penetrates the bloodstream, releasing toxic byproducts into the body. This causes many different health problems, ranging from digestive issues to depression. Most complete probiotic supplements contain Saccharomyces, a yeast which inhibits the growth of Candida, and is essential

to balancing gut flora. You will find saccharomyces as a major ingredient in immunity boosters and other probiotic supplements.

Antibiotics kill both good and bad bacteria in the gut. Bifidobacteria and acidophilus, which are beneficial probiotics in our guts, produce antifungal and antibacterial substances that balance the gut flora as well as manufacture B vitamins. When this balance is disturbed by antibiotics and other drugs, all body systems are affected. Candida requires sugar in order to grow; and the Western high-sugar diet is a predisposing factor for the epidemic of candidiasis.

Acne and Antibiotics

According to the founder of the Paleo diet, Dr. Loren Cordain, and author of *The Dietary Cure for Acne* mentioned earlier in this book, skin problems and acne are rooted in dietary sensitivities and can be the result of overuse of antibiotics which is traditional medicine's routine treatment for acne. A decade ago, Dr. Loren Cordain published his study on the Paleolithic diet, claiming that increased intestinal permeability or "Leaky Gut Syndrome" (LGS) causes body-wide inflammation, a slow "burn" that accelerates aging. Gliadin, the protein found in wheat, is a primary cause of LGS.

Dr. Cordain also identifies these substances as contributors to Leaky Gut Syndrome: milk, grains, potatoes, hot spices, alcohol, refined sugar and carbohydrates, birth control pills, antacids and other pharmaceuticals.

"Bad" gut bacteria binds to cell walls of the gut lining, causing the immune system to become inflamed. According to Dr. Cordain, chronic low-level inflammation drives heart disease, cancer, type 2 diabetes, skin conditions, GI problems, and mental disorders. Dr. Cordain recommends avoiding foods introduced since the agricultural revolution, along with processed foods and pharmaceuticals. Supplements to promote healthy gut flora is the best prevention—probiotics from fresh plants, fermented foods, and probiotics such as those found in apples and leeks.

The Impact of Roundup on Gut Health

Research scientist Dr. Stephanie Seneffat of the Massachusetts Institute of Technology explains, "In addition to aiding in digestion, gut microbiota synthesize vitamins, detoxify xenobiotics, and participate in immune system homeostasis and gastrointestinal tract permeability." Her research has found that glyphosate residue in our foods inhibits other enzymes that detox xenobiotics—other foreign chemicals in our bodies. The presence of this special herbicide has an additive toxic effect allowing other toxins to build up, but more importantly glyphosate prohibits gut bacteria from functioning. "There is a disruption of the biosynthesis of aromatic amino acids by gut bacteria," she writes. Even though the effect of glyphosate on humans cannot be directly measured, it does have a profound effect on gut bacteria producing a toxic environment which inhibits the breakdown of protein into three essential amino acids: phenylalanine, tyrosine, and tryptophan. This breakdown is part of the "shikimate pathway," which is absent in all mammals. For this reason, manufacturers of these disrupting herbicides claim that it is safe and nontoxic for humans even though we depend on our gut bacteria for synthesis of amino acids, and these bacteria are profoundly affected by exposure to herbicides.

Glyphosate and Autism

Number of children (6-21yrs) with autism served by IDEA plotted against glyphosate use on corn & soy

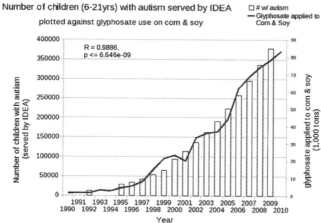

Examiner.com. Glyphosate and Neurological Disorders. www.examiner.com slideshow/gmos-glyphosate-and-neurological-disorders#slide=1.

Consider the three amino acids synthesized by gut bacteria free of herbicide exposure: Phenylalanine is a precursor for tyrosine, which is essential for thyroid and adrenal function. Low levels of tyrosine are also associated with skin aging. A study published in Behavioral and Brain Functions identifies tryptophan as deficient in children with ADHD. Dr. Johansson reported that children with ADHD have a 50 percent lower level of tryptophan, which is important for the production of serotonin, 95% of which is produced in the gut. In addition to depression, serotonin deficiency is associated with greater impulsivity, which is a core symptom of ADHD. Dr. Johansson also found changes in the cellular membrane, which affected the transport of alanine, resulting in higher levels in the brain.

Finally, in Dr. Seneff's opinion, "glyphosate may be the most significant environmental toxin, mainly because it is pervasive and is often handled carelessly due to its perceived nontoxicity." An Australian researcher from the University of Canterbury published research showing that genetically altered wheat whose genes have been "silenced" to produce lower carbohydrate content, also can "silence" human genes. Eating this wheat could lead to significant changes in the way the body stores glucose and carbohydrates and may begin to explain the high levels of obesity in America.

Since the 1990s when herbicides began to be used on food crops engineered to live through their application, various diseases and conditions have increased dramatically. Scientists are attributing the increase in digestive issues, obesity, autism, Alzheimer's disease, depression, Parkinson's disease, liver disease, cancer, and ADHD to the disruption of the gut biome. Are you ready to clean out your pantry? Read every label. Throw away wheat, corn (including high fructose corn syrup), soy (including lecithin), sugar, and canola/cottonseed/corn oil.

The Effects of Poor Gut Health

Neurological effects

Dr. Nancy Swanson, a U.S. Navy scientist with a Ph.D. in Physics has declared there is a "perfect match-up between the rise in glyphosate usage and incidence of autism." According to Dr. Swanson, in addition to the gut issues, the endocrine disrupting properties of glyphosate can lead to reproductive problems: infertility, miscarriage, birth defects, and aberrant sexual development. Fetuses, infants and children are especially susceptible because they are continually experiencing growth and hormonal changes.

Confirming Dr. Swanson's research, Dr. Seneff claims that the endocrine disrupting properties of glyphosate also lead to neurological disorders, attention deficit hyperactive disorder, autism, dementia, Alzheimer's, schizophrenia and bipolar disorder. Those most susceptible are children and the elderly.

Professor Mark Lyte of Texas Tech University Health Sciences Center has proposed increasing healthy gut bacteria such as lactobacilli and bifidobacteria to improve neurological function. Research shows that gut bacteria produce and respond to neurochemicals, which have neurological and immunological effects on the body. In the face of mounting evidence of very serious side effects to the promise of feeding a hungry world, Monsanto, the manufacturer of Roundup has petitioned the FDA and received approval to increase its residue levels of glyphosate, as weeds are becoming increasingly resistant to Roundup, creating superweeds that are resistant all together. Roundup resistant weeds have been found in 18 countries.

Creating food crops that resist pesticides has resulted in a sharp increase of chemical pesticide usage. In 2007, 1.6 billion pounds of Roundup were used in the U.S. Dow Agro Sciences has developed an entirely new generation of soybeans, corn and cotton that resist the major ingredient in "Agent Orange," an herbicide that is widely used around the world. What is new is that farmers no longer have to apply it carefully and sparingly. Food crops will withstand the herbicide, making it easy to indiscriminately dump the chemicals on food, without consideration for the resulting super-weeds or the sharp increase in the use of chemical pesticides and herbicides with significant adverse health implications.

Obesity and Inflammation

Obesity in Teenagers Has More Than Quadrupled Since 1971.

A study funded by the National Institutes of Health has identified 26 species of bacteria in the human gut microbiota that appear to be linked to obesity, inflammation, and related metabolic complications such as insulin resistance, high blood sugar levels, hypertension and high cholesterol. The researchers' sample included 310 members of the Amish community of Lancaster, Pennsylvania, because their diet and lifestyles are very similar to one another.

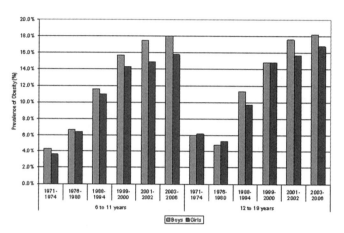

It is very easy to increase the colonies of healthy gut flora by taking supplements containing live cultures. An Irish scientist published research in the journal *Microbiology*, associating low levels of healthy gut bacteria with obesity and colon cancer. A University of Michigan study published in *Gastroenterology* showed that the effect of inflammation on the gut could be protected with probiotics, which reversed the presence of an inflammatory component. Stress inhibits the presence of these anti-inflammatories, but can be mitigated with the use of probiotics.

Some Lactobacillus species are used for the production of yogurt, cheese, sauerkraut, pickles, beer, wine, cider, kimchi, cocoa, and other fermented foods, as well as animal feeds, such as silage. Sourdough bread is made using a "starter culture," which is a symbiotic culture of yeast and lactic acid bacteria growing in a water and flour medium.

I myself am all too familiar with this inflammatory concept. While in medical school in the 90's, we were taught what at the time was believed to be good nutrition that would lower cholesterol levels and prevent heart disease. That was the cardiac, low fat diet which most people have followed since the 80's. That diet conditioned us to eat a tremendous amount of carbs. We were taught that fat was bad, and carbs were okay. As a young medical student I had all but eliminated fat from my diet in an attempt to be healthy. The problem was that I created an inflammatory environment that led to arthritis, PMS, thyroid disease, abnormal menstrual cycles, and declined cognitive abilities. All of this because I had eliminated all fat, including essential fats from my diet. Essential fats, often called Omega 3's, are supplements that everyone should be taking. They help with carbohydrate metabolism, the reduction of cholesterol/triglycerides, they are what the body uses to do repair work at the cellular level within the gut, the brain, the connective tissues and the list goes on.

Premature Birth

A double-blind Canadian research study measured weight gain in extremely low birthweight premature babies. They found that giving fifty such infants daily doses of lactobacillus and bifidobacterium resulted in better weight gain as compared with 51 infants who received no supplements, and there were no side effects from giving probiotic supplements. "These findings demonstrate the role of gut flora in nutrient absorption," according to Dr. Al-Hosni of the St. Louis University School of Medicine. An Australian study also identified probiotics as treatment for necrotizing enterocolitis, an infection which destroys the bowel lining in premature babies. Although there was no effect on the risk of infection, the risk of death was reduced by 53% in groups given probiotics.

A UCLA study has raised the question of the safety of antibiotics destroying gut bacteria in premature infants. Antibiotics are used extensively in neonatal intensive care and in child respiratory tract infections and the suppression of normal gut bacteria have long term consequences on brain development.

Anxiety/Depression

A study published in the journal *Gut Pathogens* describes thirty-nine patients with chronic fatigue syndrome who were treated with lactobacillus. Patients reported a significant reduction in anxiety compared to a group that received a placebo. This makes complete sense because our neurotransmitters, or feel good substances, like serotonin and norepinephrine are produced in the gut. When you clean up the gut, allowing the gut to function at optimal levels, you increase the production of these substances. In addition, some of those good gut bacteria play a significant role in the utilization of the amino acids tyrosine and tryptophan, both of which are precursors for serotonin production. When I have a patient presenting with mild depression or anxiety, the first thing I want to do is address the gut by cleaning up their diet and giving them a good prebiotic, probiotic and digestive enzyme. In addition, I want to make sure they have the amino acids necessary to make appropriate levels of serotonin so I often start them on 5-HTP (5-hydroxytryptophan). This gives their body the amino acid tryptophan, which is needed to make the serotonin.

Hepatic Encephalopathy and Fatty Liver

This disease is caused by an accumulation of toxins in the blood that are normally removed by the liver. Symptoms include personality change, intellectual impairment, and reduced consciousness, with a poor prognosis. Conventional treatments of laxatives and antibiotics harm the gut flora. A new study announced by the European Association for the Study of the Liver found that 160 liver patients improved significantly over a nine-month period using probiotic capsules for treatment. Fatty Liver is a condition in which the individual has elevated liver enzymes, similar to what you would see with alcoholism/liver cirrhosis. Their liver upon examination by MRI or CT is found to be encased in fat thus the term "fatty liver disease". Most doctors just watch that condition, rechecking enzymes regularly and perhaps repeating the scan yearly. The patient is usually over weight or can be of normal weight but still obese based on body fat analysis. Some people with what is referred to "normal weight" obesity, have large amounts of visceral fat or "organ fat". The fatty liver cannot function properly so the enzymes elevate. The liver can no longer do its very important body task, "detoxification". This condition can be reversed by cleaning up the gut, changing the diet to clean/whole food/low carb/good lean protein, whole body detoxification, correcting nutrient deficiencies and adding Omega 3 essential fatty acids both in the diet and as a supplement because they need the support.

Osteoporosis

The lead author of a University of Michigan study reports, "inflammation in the gut can cause bone loss, though it's unclear exactly why." Lactobacillus probiotics were fed to male mice, which showed significant increase in bone density after four weeks of treatment. This is especially significant for people with IBS and Type I Diabetes, because bone loss accompanies these conditions, and the current drugs have negative side effects.

In addition, a study conducted by the University College of Cork, Ireland found a correlation between frailty, lack of cognitive function, inflammation, poor diet and the microbiota composition from 178 elderly subjects residing in various assisted living communities. Health declined with the loss of healthy gut flora.

Inflammatory Bowel Disease and Crohn's

Researchers from the University of Michigan have concluded that it is overly simple to say that stress causes Irritable Bowel Syndrome. However, there is conclusive evidence that stress changes brain-gut interactions, which produces inflammation leading to pain, loss of appetite and diarrhea.

A study conducted at Georgia Regents University and published in the journal *Nature* found that immune diseases result from T-cells attacking the normal gut bacteria. Regulatory T-cells that keep this from happening are produced in the thymus, a hormone regulating organ near the heart. Vitamin A can aid in the maturation of T-cells to protect the gut bacteria.

Cognitive Function

A study by UCLA researchers produced evidence that beneficial bacteria in the gut enhanced by taking probiotics altered brain function in women. During the resting brain scan, there was greater connectivity between the brain stem and prefrontal cortex. The researchers are now seeking to identify the chemicals produced by gut bacteria that may trigger signals to the brain.

Aging

The journal *Nature* reports a long term study of the elderly, which found that the gut bacteria correlate significantly with problems such as frailty, inflammation, impaired cognitive function, absorption of metabolites, and decreased longevity. The data supports a relationship between diet, the presence of gut microflora, and overall health, indicating the need for diet-driven gut support to slow the health decline due to aging. Lead researcher Paul O'Toole said he was surprised by "the correlation between gut microbiota and the health of older people."

Bruising and Clotting Issues

Hemorrhaging under the skin may indicate a deficiency of Vitamin K, which is a byproduct of bacterial metabolism.

Autoimmune Disease

It has long been known that there is a direct correlation between autoimmune diseases and what is going on within the gut. There is a very clear association of autoimmune thyroid disease and gluten sensitivity. Many notable physicians and experts recommend those with autoimmune diseases should follow a gluten free diet. Seventy to 90 percent of the immune system actually resides within the gut. If the gut is not functioning at optimal levels, then the immune system is not functioning at optimal levels either.

Food Is Absorbed as Information

Betty Crocker Carrot Cake Mix (a product of General Mills) is actually a carrot-free product, with "carrot flavored pieces" cooked up from corn syrup, flour, corn cereal, harmful partially hydrogenated cottonseed or soybean oil (likely from genetically engineered crops), and artificial colors Yellow 6 and Red 40.

Obesity, diabetes, depression, heart disease and irritable bowel syndrome are but a handful of conditions that may be helped by rebalancing your gut flora. Over 30 different beneficial pharmacological actions of probiotics have been identified and more than 200 studies show probiotics can be helpful for over 170 diseases. Symptoms indicating you're lacking healthy bacteria include gas, bloating, constipation, frequent nausea, headaches, and sugar cravings.

Finally, Pollan in *Cooked* describes the ever present tug, "in life, of death." All of plants and animals carry an invisible world of microbes ready to set up decomposition. These microbes carry the enzymes necessary to reduce intricate molecular life structures into food the microbes can consume. Sturdy cellular walls constructed of cellulose or lignin, carbohydrates too complex for most microbes to penetrate, protect plants from microbial decomposition and for humans skin, a larger system of epithelial cells hold most bugs at bay. In the gut a gastrointestinal skin protected by a layer of carbohydrate rich mucus provides a barrier to the microbes. Ah the cycle of life, decay and reuse through fermentation and it can all taste so good and be helpful to gut health. Previous generations tied to land instead of cities received the yield from the fields and preserved a quality of it by fermentation. Today much of the understanding and technique of fermenting is lost to us and also lost are the wonderful and unique flavors and most importantly the nourishment for the body and also the gut.

How to Improve Your Gut Health

- **Enzyme and Probiotic Supplements**

  A youthful healthy gut produces digestive enzymes such as pepsin, protease, amylase, and lipase, to break down food into the amino acids necessary for healthy metabolism. As a person ages, these enzymes, which are dependent on the pancreas, decrease, resulting in less than optimal digestion of foods. Probiotic bacteria are the digestion factory in the gut. The common probiotics such as lactobacillus are not as effective, since they do not survive the strong acidic environment of the stomach. Unlike lactobacillus, the majority of Bacillus coagulans survives and thrives in the gut.

  Green algae Chlorella enhances growth and multiplication of probiotics by a factor of four. It contains abundant protein and chlorophyll and all of the essential amino acids, and has been used to treat symptoms of anxiety in people with chronic fatigue.

  What about yogurt? Manufacturers of processed yogurt expose the finished product to high heat in order to shut down fermentation, which kills the bacteria, but gives the yogurt a longer shelf life. The dry probiotic enzymes will survive the stomach's acid, because they are designed to bypass it, and become active in the intestine. Yogurt may help with constipation and give a sense of benefit because it contains a potent laxative, inulin. It is a filler and stabilizer used in processed foods, and keeps dairy products from separating. However, this yogurt product is doing nothing to enhance the gut microflora, which affects every health system.

  A good prebiotic is a fiber that is fermented in the large intestine, and provides nourishment for the probiotic bacteria to proliferate. Examples are inulin and oligofructose. These stimulate the production of good bacteria in the colon, and help to stabilize blood sugar, cholesterol, and triglycerides. Most probiotic supplements contain live cultures of different species of Lactobacillus and Bifidobacteria.

  Most of us have allowed wheat gluten to create intestinal "road rash". It has damaged the intestinal microvilli, interfering with absorption of key nutrients as well as detoxification of the body. In the case of the gut, if you give the body what it needs, it can often repair itself. Give your gut a good prebiotic, probiotic and digestive enzyme.

- **Eliminate Inflammation**

  Belly fat is unique in the way it triggers inflammation. It is a metabolic factory, and as it increases, it causes abnormal insulin responses, diabetes, hypertension and heart disease, dementia, rheumatoid arthritis, and colon cancer. Citing to the Proceedings of the Japan Academy of Physiology and Biological Science, Dr. Davis explains that your belly fat acts like an endocrine gland producing abnormal inflammatory signals that are released into the bloodstream (p. 62). Belly fat is a factory for estrogen production in both sexes. Estrogen stimulates the growth of breast tissue, and increases the incidence of breast cancer. Inflammation can be significantly reduced by repairing the gut with prebiotics, probiotics and digestive enzymes, by adding Omega 3 essential fats, by eating a whole food/clean diet and eating low glycemic index foods which will in turn help to keep insulin levels low.

- **Maintain Healthy Blood Glucose Levels**

  Americans could accurately be described as wheat-a-holics, with a per capita consumption of 133 pounds of wheat annually. This equals a half loaf of bread per day. Wheat pushes blood sugar higher than other foods. When the cycle of glucose-insulin reaches abnormal highs and lows several times a day, it provokes growth of belly fat, which is associated with insulin resistance, which leads to even higher levels of glucose and insulin, damaging pancreatic beta cells, and making the wheat addict more susceptible to diabetes.

  Wheat consumption is also associated with bone calcium depletion. Osteoporosis is associated with chronic acidosis in the body, causing calcium to be taken from the bones to balance the body's pH at 7.4. In young people the most obvious pH disrupter comes from carbonated drinks loaded with carbonic acid and phosphoric acid. Calcium salts from the bones are drawn into the blood and tissues to neutralize an acid challenge. A constant acidic environment stimulates bone-reabsorbing cells, osteoclasts, to work harder and faster to dissolve bone tissue and release calcium. Wheat is among the most potent sources of sulfuric acid, yielding more per gram than meat. Grains account for 38 percent of the acid load in the average American. Meat also renders the body more acidic and should be balanced by alkaline vegetables. Wheat tips the scale to a chronic acid load on the body, driving the body to deplete bone calcium. The money for osteoporosis drugs now exceeds $10 billion a year.

- **Eat Fermented Foods**

  Fermenting is ancient and specific to a particular locale as plants and animals are taken from an area to produce a preserve – a food that is available for consumption after harvested. Today we understand this cooking process the least, but coffee, cheese, olives, kimchi, kefir, sour dough, sour milk, chocolate, vanilla, bread, cheese, wine, beer, yogurt, ketchup and most other condiments depend upon fermentation. There are lactic-acid ferments, alkaline ferments and alcohol ferments from cultures all over the world. Giving a nod to "fermentos" Gregor Reid from the University of Western Ontario recommends microbial strains found in fermented foods as especially beneficial for producing neurochemicals. (*BioEssays*, July 2011)

- **Omega 3 Essential Fatty Acid Supplement**

  Omega 3's are a supplement that everyone should be taking. In the gut, they help with the absorption of carbs, they are used to repair gaps that occur between cells from damage caused by gluten, and they help stabilize blood sugar levels, which in turn keeps insulin levels low. In addition, they decrease the amount of beta amyloid protein build up in the brain. Beta amyloid is the protein that causes "tangles" in the brain and leads to Alzheimer's disease. Studies show that Omega 3's reduce the amount of beta amyloid protein. 1000mg can reduce the beta amyloid by 30%, 2000mg can reduce by 60%. This supplement is one of the first I use to address cognitive issues.

- **Correct Nutrient Deficiencies**

  If your gut is not functioning properly, you are not absorbing food and nutrients. On top of that you probably are not even able to get all the nutrients your body needs from our current food supply. Correcting nutrient deficiencies can make huge improvements in overall health. For example, if an individual has hypertension and they also are deficient in vitamin D (most of us are), they can see as much as an 8mm of mercury decrease in their blood pressure, just from correcting their Vitamin D deficiency. Taking a good multi vitamin that is specifically developed for maximum absorption is key. This is the single best way to correct nutritional deficiencies that you may not even be aware exist.

- **Avoid GMO Food**

  Finally avoid the GMO quartet—read every label, and do not buy any product that contains corn, soy, sugar, or canola/cottonseed oil. Buying organic foods is the right solution. When eliminating genetically modified food and buying organic foods, you are avoiding pesticide sprays, antibiotics in meat, and unnecessary chemical additives that create a toxic store in your body depriving you of optimal health.

Chapter 3 Recommendations

- Eat a clean organic diet of fresh or frozen meat and vegetables
- Avoid wheat, processed and GMO food, balance hormones to eliminate belly fat
- Replace sugar with natural stevia. Occasional sugar consumption should be limited to organic cane sugar, never beet sugar (which is GM).
- Favor low glycemic index foods
- Avoid antibiotics, including meat from injected animals. Use colloidal silver and D-mannose as natural alternatives
- Supplement with high quality digestive enzymes, prebiotics and probiotics
- Cleanse your blood and major organs with a detoxification treatment
- Supplement with Omega 3's for brain health

Chapter 4
Metabolic Syndrome

Metabolic Syndrome is the combination of insulin resistance (type 2 diabetes), hypertension and high cholesterol. The combination of these three conditions accelerates the aging of every organ system in the body and dramatically decreases optimal body function. It leads to adrenal stress, and imbalance of hormones throughout the body. It is strongly implicated in polycystic ovarian disease (PCOS), coronary artery disease, and higher overall morbidity (disease) and mortality (death) rates.

Insulin Resistance

If you lack energy, wonder often if you're "coming down with something," and fight fatigue every day, you may be struggling with insulin resistance. Insulin resistance occurs when cells fail to respond to the hormone insulin. This happens when the body has been forced to produce a large amount of insulin in response to continuous, on-going high glycemic load, which is caused by eating too much sugar and refined carbs and the system eventually wears down and then out! Insulin resistance (IR) rides along for years wearing down energy and productivity levels. IR has increased dramatically in the past 10 years, rising along with the rates of metabolic syndrome in the U.S.

Metabolic syndrome can be signaled by fogginess and inability to focus; high blood sugar; intestinal bloating (most intestinal gas is produced from carbohydrates that humans do not digest and absorb well), sleepiness especially after meals, weight gain, fat storage, and difficulty losing weight (excess weight is from high fat storage). The fat of insulin resistance is generally stored in and around abdominal organs in both males and females and it is likely that hormones produced in that fat are a precipitating cause of insulin resistance, increased blood triglyceride levels, and increased blood pressure. Three out of four Americans today are either overweight or obese, and a staggering thirty percent of U.S. children are also overweight or obese.

Due to the deranged metabolism resulting from insulin resistance, psychological effects, including depression, are not uncommon. Making this all more difficult: levels of hunger – literally feeding the problem – rise. Though it is complicated by a number of malfunctioning systems, this common condition, Metabolic Syndrome, can in many cases be reversed through diet, nutrient supplementation, and exercise.

The role of insulin is to regulate the delivery of glucose into the cells for storage allowing the glucose to provide energy to the cell or be stored for later utilization by the body. Cells that are resistant to insulin can't take in glucose, fatty acids or amino acids. This causes glucose, fatty acids and amino acids to leak out of the cell, further elevating the circulating levels within the blood stream.

According to an article in The New England Journal of Medicine, it is estimated 91 percent of diabetes could be prevented if people followed a low glycemic diet (low carbs and sugars) and got 30 minutes of vigorous exercise daily. (N Eng J Med 2001;(11):790-797). Again, the solution is literally at the end of our forks in most cases!

Hypertension

In medical school I learned an ideal blood pressure goal, which was an arbitrary number below 120/80. Every patient should ideally have a blood pressure in this range, and those who didn't needed treatment. It didn't really matter how you solved the problem, you just did it, often putting the patient on multiple anti hypertensives that had numerous side effects as well as many drug interactions. Finding the right combination was often daunting. Dr. Mark Houston of Vanderbilt University has written an excellent book on hypertension, which I highly recommend if you or someone you love has hypertension. He has also written a medical textbook on the topic. In his book, *What Your Doctor May Not Tell You About Hypertension,* he helps people understand the factors that play into this disease as well as the silent damage that takes place for those who have it.

Hypertension is a manifestation of the health of the blood vessel. If a blood vessel is healthy then the blood pressure will be at or below 115/70. When the blood pressure starts to creep above that number it is an indication that there is inflammation, oxidative stress and most likely an autoimmune-like state taking place within the lining of the blood vessel.

People with hypertension are often either diabetic or pre-diabetic and have elevated insulin levels due to insulin resistance. One of insulin's jobs is to control arterial wall tension throughout the body, and a lack of elasticity in the arterial walls will increase blood pressure. Cytokines are regulatory proteins, which communicate between cells to promote immunity. There is an abnormal level of pro-inflammatory cytokines released from fat cells, which contributes to insulin resistance, cardiovascular disease and rheumatoid arthritis. When insulin levels are corrected, there is dramatic improvement in the other two components of metabolic syndrome as well.

As diseased blood vessels begin to lose elasticity, blood pressure numbers begin to escalate. Think of it this way: Imagine the different rate at which water flows through a flexible garden hose versus the rate of flow through a steel pipe. If you were to apply the same amount of water pressure at the entry point of the flexible hose and the rigid metal pipe, the rigid metal pipe would have much higher pressure at the ending point, and it's much the same with blood vessels. As the blood vessel becomes stiff and rigid, blood pressure numbers increase.

Misunderstanding in medicine has led to the mistreatment of hypertension. As it is now better understood, it makes sense to determine exactly what it is that is causing the inflammation in the blood vessels (which is also causing inflammation throughout the body), or what is causing oxidative stress along the lining of the vessels, or what is causing an autoimmune reaction along the lining of the vessels. When the actual cause is determined, it is often possible to see dramatic improvements in the health of the blood vessel, which are indeed measurable, as well as improvements in the rest of the body. Remember blood vessels are the body's transportation system and, if they are sick, the entire body is operating below optimum levels or sick!

Treating the blood vessel starts with a diet high in protein and complex carbohydrates, all low on the glycemic index. There are many supplements that can make a dramatic difference as well. Many supplements act like natural calcium channel blockers or even ACE inhibitors. Both of these are blood pressure medications. The ones proven in studies to be of benefit are: Vitamins B6, B12, C and E, CoEnzyme Q10, Folic Acid, L-Arginine, Garlic and Alpha Lipoic Acid.

High Cholesterol

The third element of metabolic syndrome is high cholesterol, high triglycerides or a variation thereof. For a long time medicine has also treated patients using test numbers without fully understanding the process or disease behind it. It turns out that a person can have completely normal total cholesterol, normal LDL (the bad cholesterol) and a healthy amount of HDL (the good cholesterol), BUT they can still have coronary artery disease! It seems it is more important to look at the number of LDL particles in the blood (the less the better) and the size of the LDL particles (the bigger the better) because this is what determines the likelihood of these particles crossing the damaged lining of the blood vessel and setting up plaque formation. This measurement can be assessed with an expanded lipid panel, a blood test now offered through most labs. We used to think the higher the HDL numer the better, but now we know that the quality of HDL matters too. Larger HDL is actually better because it is able to transport a lot of the LDL particles away! HDL functions as a transport mechanism or a clean up crew.

The following supplements have been recommended to lower cholesterol: Garlic, ginseng, fenugreek, high soluble fiber, Omega 3's, EPA and DPA (fish oil), niacin, and red yeast rice.

Aspartame and MSG

A 2008 study at the University of Minnesota linked diet soda to metabolic syndrome. According to the study, consuming diet drinks increase the risk of developing metabolic syndrome by 34 percent. Aspartame, also known as NutraSweet or Equal, was approved for use in food in 1981, and is the sweetener used in diet drinks and most diet food. It was developed by G. D. Searle Pharmaceuticals, a company purchased by Monsanto in 1983. Aspartame accounts for over 75 percent of adverse reactions to food additives reported to the FDA. Aspartame and MSG act in the body as neurotransmitters, and an overabundance destroys neurons by triggering free radicals, which kill the cells. Because we use only a small portion of our brain cells, a large majority of cells must be damaged in a particular area before symptoms are present. However researchers have found a correlation between aspartame consumption and migraine headaches, fatigue, depression, and memory loss. Aspartame should be avoided in light of the huge spike in neurological disease—multiple sclerosis, Alzheimer's disease, brain cancer, Parkinson's disease, and dementia.

Fasting

Research studies over the past decade suggest that intermittent fasting could reduce the risk of cancer, guard against diabetes and heart disease, help control asthma, and improve brain function while protecting against Parkinson's disease and dementia. A fast starts 10 to 12 hours after the last meal when all of the available glucose in the blood is used up, and the liver begins to convert glycogen and fat to usable energy. The liver produces ketones in the process, which can be used by the brain for fuel. At the Longevity Institute at the University of Southern California, short term fasts were found to slow the growth of five of eight cancer tumors in animals. Dr. Stephen Freedland of Duke University claims that "undernutrition without malnutrition" is the only experimental approach that improves survival in animals with cancer.

A 24 hour, once-a-month water only fast will raise the level of human growth hormone, which triggers the breakdown of fat, and reduces insulin levels. According to The American Journal of Cardiology, this reduces the risk of diabetes and coronary heart disease. Human Growth Hormone is also elevated in other fasting plans, such as limiting your eating to an eight hour window each day (Dr. Mercola recommends 11:00 a.m. to 7:00 p.m.), or the "5:2" fasting plan where two days a week you eat a single meal of less than 600 calories.

Mark Mattson of the NIH Institute on Aging recommends alternate day fasting, where you eat a single meal under 600 calories every other day. He found that after a few weeks, asthma symptoms improved, and inflammation markers decreased. He found that fasting increases brain activity, and boosts the production of a brain protein called brain-derived neurotropic factor by 50 to 400 percent. This protein stimulates the generation of new brain cells and plays a role in learning and memory. It protects brain cells from changes associated with Alzheimer's and Parkinson's. He also found a reduction in insulin resistance.

Fasting causes your body to shift from burning sugar and carbs to burning fat as its primary fuel. Once your body has made this shift, cravings for sugar and food in general will radically decrease. From the third day onward, the breakdown of fat continues to increase, peaking on the tenth day. The heightened state of ketosis is similar to sleep when the body rests and detoxes. Energy that was focused on digestion can be redirected to immunity and detoxification. Toxins are stored in fat cells, so as these cells are broken down, the toxins are released and can be eliminated through the liver. Replacement of damaged cells occurs more efficiently. This is why animals may stop eating when they are wounded, and why humans are often not hungry when plagued with a fever.

In a clinical trial to reduce hypertension, 174 people ate only fruits and vegetables for three days, then participated in a 10 day water only fast, followed by a week of low fat vegan diet. Ninety percent of the participants achieved blood pressure less than 140/90 by the end of the trial. The average drop for all participants was 37/13, and those with severe hypertension had an average reduction of 60/17. A fasting lifestyle could be a major tool in overcoming our current epidemic of Metabolic Syndrome in America.

If you feel overwhelmed by the changes you need to make because your health profile is so complex, you will be encouraged by Gary Kehoe's story. In about eight months he reversed a health crisis, amazing family, friends and his doctors!

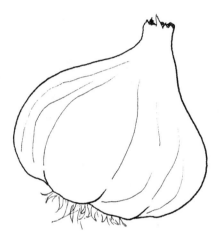

Treating Metabolic Syndrome with Nutrition
By Gary Kehoe

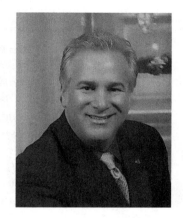

As a diabetic patient at the Columbus Veterans Hospital, I was having my liver function tested before my doctor prescribed a cholesterol medicine (my LDL was over 125, and they wanted it below 100). On Jan 17, 2012, a blood test was done to test liver function, and my readings were ALT 125 and AST 37. I was told those were way too high to tolerate any medication and they would retest me in a couple months when I returned from a business trip.

I was retested on March 21, 2012 and my readings were ALT 144, AST 42, ALKPHOS 54, TBILI 0.45. Again I was told my readings were way too high for any cholesterol medication, and my liver was not good. Worst of all, if things didn't improve I was facing liver failure. Once again, they would retest after I returned from my next business trip (I was constantly away on trips lasting from 4-5 weeks).

After I returned a few months later, I was referred to a GI doctor and she had an ultra sound test done to see if I had fatty liver syndrome. All of the images did not show any fatty liver, so I was tested again for liver function on Sept 24, 2012, and my readings were even worse: ALT 186, AST 64, ALKPHOS 62, TBILI 0.55, DBILI 0.12. Again I was leaving on another string of business trips, so the GI doctor said that the next time she saw me in December, she wanted me to lose 20 pounds to see if that helped, and we would test again and go from there.

While I was on a trip at the end of September, one of the people in the office I was working at in Illinois gave me a sample of protein powder, detox tea, and appetite curbing chews (as I told her I needed to lose some weight). When I got back to Columbus the second week of November, I found someone who sold the protein supplement, and started on a full weight loss program that eliminated gluten, dairy, sugar, and bad oils. I began the program with a seven day detox, and entered the holiday season determined to work the plan. I started the 30-day fitness plan the day before Thanksgiving…. Not an easy task!! Needless to say, I followed the plan to a "T" and lost 20 pounds by Christmas. Two vegan protein shakes a day, Detox Tea daily, no dairy, no coffee, and I reduced meat intake to only once or twice a week. The protein supplement provided a 100 percent amino acid profile, so I didn't need to eat high fat meat, which is loaded with calories and taxes the liver.

By the time I saw my doctor on January 8, 2013, I was down 25 pounds, and she was ecstatic!! I said, "you told me to lose 20 pounds so I did." She said she tells patients to lose weight every day, and no one ever does, or if they do, it's only a few pounds, and I had exceeded her goal. She was so pleased, and even more amazed when my liver function blood test results came back: ALT 71, AST 26, ALKPHOS 67, TBILI 0.46, DBILI 0.10. She could not believe that I had dropped over 100 points in such a short period of time. When I told her what I had been eating and supplementing, she said, "keep it up!" She tested me again on January 25, 2013, and again my results dropped: ALT 66, AST 28, ALKPHOS 68, TBILI 0.52. She said I was still a little high, but was out of any danger. She would see me in 3 months. My regular doctor also did some blood on the Jan 25th, My A1C was down to 6.2 (from 6.5), my LDL was down to 112 from over 125.

During this time, I was also on Lisinopril for Hypertension, 20mg a day, but my Blood Pressure was consistently low (110 over 65on average). My doctor reduced my dosage to 10mg. I was also on 1000mg of Metformin for my diabetes, but that wasn't changed.

When I went back to the GI doctor on April 5, 2013, my liver function tests were ALT 54, AST 25, ALKPHOS 57, TBILI 0.50, DBILI 0.08. She was truly amazed at my progress, and that my readings were within normal ranges!! She said she would see me in two years. My regular doctor also tested me again for cholesterol, and my LDL was now down to 93. He was very excited because I had dropped my cholesterol by over 30 points. Also my blood pressure was still staying at a steady 110 over 65 even after the dosage being cut in half from 20mg to 10mg, so he reduced it again to 5mg a day.

On my last visit to my regular doctor on August 13, 2013, my A1C was down to 6.0!!! Very exciting, down from 6.5! Also my blood pressure was still steady at 110 over 65, so he once again reduced my Lisinopril from 5mg to 2.5mg a day. That is a reduction from 20mg to 2.5mg in just over 6 months. He still won't reduce my Metformin dosage, said we'll see when I see him in 6 months....

I'd like to be able to say that all of this changed because I became active, hit the gym every day, exercised all the time, etc., but I didn't. Yes I do try to walk once or twice a week, but that's about all I have time for. I went from being on the edge of liver failure to being completely normal in less than 6 months!!! I reduced my LDL cholesterol over 30 points in the same period. I reduced my BP med dosage from 20mg to 2.5mg in just over 8 months. AND I lost a total of 40 pounds, and all I did was change my nutritional intake to clean, healthy foods and supplements. I can't say nutrition "cured" my issues, but the ONLY thing I *changed in my life was to clean up my diet, use a total body seven day cleanse, and drink the Detox Tea almost daily.*

To this day, I still have two protein shakes a day, and drink my tea. I'm still down 40 pounds, and I have MY LIFE BACK!! I can't begin to describe how scared I was when the doctor said I was on the edge of liver failure (cirrhosis) if things didn't improve. For me, this past year was truly a year of PURE TRANSFORMATION!!!!

2012
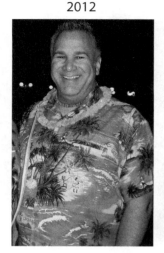

2013
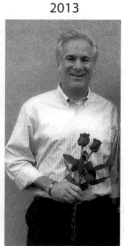

Chapter 4 Recommendations:

- Diet high in protein and complex carbohydrates with a low glycemic index
- Avoid grains, especially wheat and soy
- Walking, daily moderate exercise
- Natural supplements that strengthen blood vessel walls and lower cholesterol
- A regular fasting regimen

Chapter 5
The Neurological Impact of Nutritionally Depleted Foods & Toxins

The neurological benefits of good nutrition are, like gut health, a new field in the research spotlight. This chapter will examine completed studies as well as research in progress that points to a correlation between nutrition and neurological health. Some studies included here are inconclusive, but it is significant that researchers can no longer ignore the skyrocketing statistics for brain cancer, Alzheimer's, Parkinson's, Autism, and other neurological diseases that were rare a generation ago.

In 1954, Dr. Denham Harmon proposed that aging and disease can trace its genesis to the effects of free radicals. Today his theory is accepted as the best explanation of the aging process, and the cellular damage associated with dementia, Alzheimer's, stroke, arthritis, autoimmune diseases, and cancer. Because of our exponential exposure to processed food, (the average American eats 100 pounds of trans-fat annually), other food additives, pesticides, herbicides, chemical solvents, pharmaceuticals, water pollutants, and radiation, our bodies are overloaded with free radicals. These molecules are unstable fragments with an unpaired electron needing to accept another electron to stabilize, and having high energy levels, which have the ability to break through cell membranes, destroy enzymes, and fracture our DNA. The cell membrane is vulnerable to free radical attack because it is composed of easily oxidized (the term for accepting an electron thus stabilizing the free radical) fatty acids. The damaged membrane no longer promotes the proper transport of nutrients, oxygen and water, as well as the elimination of waste.

When a free radical breaks the DNA molecule, abnormal replication can occur which leads to cancer. Prolonged exposure to free radicals accelerates the aging process and makes us more vulnerable to disease. We must neutralize the free radicals our bodies are fighting with natural antioxidants from fresh organic fruits and vegetables, and with antioxidant enzymes, which are manufactured by healthy gut flora. Antioxidants are electron donors, and are able to neutralize free radical molecules.

Autism

Air pollution contains methylene chloride, mercury, manganese, diesel, and other particulates, which cause physical and neurological anomalies in the developing fetus. A study published in June 2013, is based on data beginning in 1989 of 116,430 nurses. From these, data on 325 women who gave birth to children with autistic spectrum symptoms and 22,000 others who did not were analyzed. Women living with the most diesel particulates and mercury have a 20% higher risk of having a child with autism. Those exposed to the highest levels of lead, methylene chloride, manganese, and heavy metals had a 50% higher risk of autism in offspring. According to the CDC, Autism spectrum disorders have increased one thousand percent in four decades. A 2010 study found that ASD is twice as likely if the mother lived within one thousand feet of a freeway during pregnancy.

A February 2013 study reported that children with autism had higher levels of lead, thallium, tin, and tungsten in their blood and urine. These are toxic metals that can impair brain development and function.

In another study published in The International Journal of Developmental Neuroscience (April, 2012), autism was associated with a deficiency of cytokines, which are small proteins released by cells of the immune system.

A study published in Clinical Epigenetics in April 2012, cited a 78% increase in autism spectrum disorder between 2002 and 2008 amongst eight year olds. This study examines the impact of High Fructose Corn Syrup on children, which is associated with the dietary loss of zinc. Zinc insufficiency negatively affects the body's ability to eliminate heavy metals, which in turn has adverse effects on young children's brain development. Consumption of HFCS also promotes loss of calcium, which aggravates the impact of lead exposure on fetuses and children. Calcium depletion also debilitates the body's ability to get rid of organophosphates, which furthers toxic effects on young brains. The researchers concluded that individual dietary factors must be considered in light of their cumulative and synergistic potential to disrupt normal development.

A research study by Kaiser Permanente of Northern California examined medical records of 1,600 children, 298 of whom had autism spectrum disorder. They found the risk doubled when mothers took SSRI antidepressants the year before birth, and was four times higher in women who took SSRI's during the first trimester. SSRI's include Prozac, Zoloft, Paxil and Celexa.

Preparing for Pregnancy:
"If only I knew then, what I know now."
with Maureen McDonnell

Maureen McDonnell has been a holistic, nutritionally-oriented pediatric registered nurse for 36 years. She is the former national coordinator of the Defeat Autism Now! Conferences and is the co-founder of children's green health expos and website: Saving Our Kids, Healing Our Planet. Her published articles include *What Can Be Done to Prevent Autism Now!*, and *Safer Ways to Vaccinate*. They can be accessed at www.SOKHOP.com. Maureen is the medical coordinator of the Imus Ranch for Kids with Cancer in New Mexico.

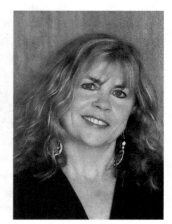

Maureen works with children that have health and developmental problems, and she has witnessed the huge effort it takes on the part of parents to improve their child's condition, once they've developed a disorder. Of course, not all illnesses are preventable, but Maureen often hears parents who are working hard to address their child's physical or behavioral issues comment, "if I only knew then, what I know now, I would have made different choices."

Something has changed. Today 1 in 6 children are affected by either a neurological, behavioral or developmental disorder. One in 50 of our kids are developing autism, asthma has tripled in the last 2 decades, 11 million children have been diagnosed with ADD and 1 in 7 of our school-aged children receive psychiatric medication.

What can be done? Maureen is adamant. It is time to consider the mother's health and wellbeing before conception more closely. After years of dedicated service helping parents and their kids achieve their full potential and attain the best possible health outcome, she believes in parents doing all possible to prevent these conditions and diseases.

The hope and promise is simple: Yes, there are no guarantees in life, but if a mother and father can optimize health prior to conceiving, they can maximize their chances of carrying, birthing, and raising a child unencumbered by ill health. Maureen is part of a growing contingent of medical professionals like Environmental and Occupational doctor Alan Liebermann of Charleston, South Carolina, who says the most important time of your life, is your mother's health the one hundred days before you are conceived. Then there is natural birth advocate Tasha Murphy:

> *Approximately 50 percent of pregnancies are unplanned, but for the remainder of babies who are consciously conceived, couples cannot underestimate their ability to influence the health of their future child. Since decades of research have shown us that certain lifestyle choices (including optimal nutrition and avoiding toxic chemicals) directly influence the health of the male and female reproductive system as well as the health of the baby, it is to a couple's advantage to educate themselves on what those lifestyle factors are, and make the necessary changes. It may be the greatest gift you give your children.*

Most of us understand poor nutrition, tobacco use, environmental toxins, STDs, alcohol, drugs etc. can pose a threat to the child's healthy development, but often left out of the mix and as significant as alcohol and smoking is the health status of the mother (and father to a degree) prior to becoming pregnant.

Babies who develop abnormal gut flora are left with compromised immune systems, and this may be a crucial factor when it comes to vaccine-induced damage. As Dr. Natasha Campbell-McBride explained in a recent interview, vaccinations were originally developed for children with healthy immune systems, and children with abnormal gut flora and therefore compromised immunity are not suitable candidates for our current vaccine schedule as they're more prone to being harmed. Another detail that helps explain how abnormal gut flora can impact your neurological status is that certain probiotics also appear to play a role in detoxing harmful chemicals.

- Dr. Mercola

Why do we need to be concerned? Unlike just a generation ago, today the impact of environmental concerns, depleted soils (poor nutrition) and discussions of "toxic burden" are often discussed and considered for what effect they may have on our health as individuals, but not necessarily when we are contemplating parenthood. Health professionals like Maureen suggest that it is possible and imperative to tip the scales in favor of having the healthiest child possible, so it just makes sense for both parents to be in an optimal state of health prior to conceiving.

In the 1980s, Maureen taught childbirth classes and worked in Labor and Delivery. Then the false belief was that the placenta protected the fetus from exposure to these toxins – many known to be carcinogenic. We now know that is not the case. The protections of the placenta are overrated due to the very porous blood brain barrier and the exposure pound for pound is greater than for those of adults.

An answer Maureen says lies in minimizing exposure to toxic substances by greening your homes and lives and laying an optimal nutritional foundation prior to conceiving. She says "give me your body for one year prior to getting pregnant, and I may be able to save you from the heartache and stress that so many parents of sick or disabled children know only too well." She addresses nutrition, removing toxic substances and heavy metals such as mercury, lead or aluminum, and assesses whether or not an overgrowth of candida or some other intestinal pathogen might be wreaking havoc on the prospective parent's health.

Maureen suggests implementing a naturally-based, nutritional approach that may include dietary changes, supplementation and a detoxification program, weight control and management, Vitamin D and Omega 3s, limiting vaccines, and in general a health overhaul. Her goal for her daughters (and for all young women in their child bearing years) is to have them be in an optimal stateof health prior to conceiving, so they can increase the likelihood of having a uncomplicated pregnancy, labor, birth and the healthiest baby possible!

For more information: www.safeminds.org/getting-healthy-before-getting-pregnant/

Dementia and Alzheimer's

New studies are examining the effects of diet on dementia, with consistent results. A September 2012 study showed decreased antioxidants, beta-carotene and vitamin C in 74 patients diagnosed with Alzheimer's, as compared to 158 matched controls, with an average age of 78.9 years. A 2010 study recommends large doses of B-complex vitamins to reduce the rate of brain shrinkage, and a February 2008 study published in the *Journal of Neurology, Neurosurgery, and Psychiatry* found that lower levels of folate can be associated with a 300 percent increased risk for dementia.

The Journal *Neurology* published a study of 1,017 individuals that compared blood glucose levels in dementia patients. They found that people whose blood sugar remains high two hours after a meal have a higher dementia risk, and those with a diagnosis of diabetes had double the risk of developing dementia. A similar study published in 2006 in the Journal of *Nutrition, Health, and Aging* found that each 1 percent increase in glycosated hemoglobin (a glucose molecule bound to the oxygen-bearing protein in red blood cells) was associated with a 40 percent increased risk of developing dementia four years later.

Both Alzheimer's and diabetes were linked to increased levels of nitrates in our environment and food in a study published in July 2009 in the *Journal of Alzheimer's Disease*. There were strong parallels between Alzheimer's, Parkinson's, and diabetes and the progressive human exposure to nitrates, nitrites and nitrosamines through processed foods and fertilizers. The authors are confident that environmental exposure plays a critical role in these insulin-resistant diseases because the rapid increase in incidence cannot be explained by mutation or other genetic change. Alzheimer's deaths have increased 150-fold from 1968 to 2005. Fertilizer consumption increased 230 percent between 1955 and 2005. Sales from fast food and meat processing increased 8 fold from 1970 to 2005, and grain consumption increased 5-fold. "We have become a nitrosamine generation," says the lead researcher. We consume processed foods, and are further exposed by nitrosamines in our food supply by leeching from the soil and contaminating water used for crop irrigation, food processing, and drinking. More than 90 percent of these compounds have been determined to be carcinogenic. Major food exposure comes from fried bacon, ground beef, cured meats, beer, and water, and non-food sources include fertilizers, pesticides, and cosmetics.

Parkinson's Disease

A study connecting pesticide exposure with Parkinson's was conducted at the Harvard School of Public Health. Data came from the 1982 American Cancer Society database of 143,325 participants. The researchers contacted 413 participants who developed Parkinson's more than ten years later, and found a 70 percent higher incidence of Parkinson's among those exposed to pesticides vs. those with no exposure.

Another article in the January 26, 2005 issue of *JAMA* linked Parkinson's disease to exposure to pesticides. At the Mayo Clinic in Rochester, Minnesota, Dr. Walter Rocca reported growing evidence that the brain is rich in estrogen, and the basal ganglia, the brain region hit hard in Parkinson's, is filled with estrogen receptors. Based on his study of 2,500 women who had their ovaries removed, premenopausal women had twice the rate of Parkinson's as those who had both their ovaries in tact.[6]

A 2011 study from the Washington University School of Medicine in St. Louis conducted a small study of 20 welders who were in good health, 20 non-welders who had Parkinson's, and 20 welders who had Parkinson's. The welders had an average of 30,000 hours of lifetime welding exposure, and their blood levels of manganese were found to be two times the upper limits of normal. Manganese has been linked to

---

6   Removing ovaries before menopause may increase risk of brain diseases. Newsday, reported in the Louisville Courier-Journal, May 1, 2005, p. A-21.

neurological problems even at low levels, and chronic exposure leads to permanent nervous system damage.

A May 2011 study of 8,534 twins in Sweden showed that individuals who are overweight during middle age are 80% more likely to develop dementia, Alzheimer's disease or vascular dementia during old age. Another study by the Boston University School of Medicine studying 733 participants associated abdominal fat in middle-aged people with lower total brain volume and dementia 30 years later. A similar study published in the journal, *Neurology* in 2008, associated waist circumference or central obesity to 2.3 times higher risk of developing dementia.

A study from Finland and Sweden followed 1,400 people for 20 years, and found that those who drink three to five cups of coffee per day in their midlife years were 65 percent less likely to develop dementia.

Bioidentical hormone balance is important for overall health, but has a particular function in neurological health. A neuroscientist at the University of South Carolina found that plant-based estrogens [phytoestrogens] are found in cells in the brain, and when these compounds are present, they slow down the cell death associated with neurodegenerative diseases such as Alzheimer's and Parkinson's Diseases. The author remarks that the use of phytoestrogens "may be novel in Western culture, but it has been used in Eastern cultures for a long time."

Vitamin D and B-12 deficiencies have been linked to Parkinson's and hand tremors. A 2009 report in the *Archives of Internal Medicine* states that as many as 77 percent of Americans are Vitamin D deficient. A 2010 study published in *Neuropsychobiology* concluded that Vitamin D supplements might reduce the symptoms of neurological disorders such as Parkinson's disease. Tremors can also be related to Vitamin B-12 deficiency, as this vitamin is essential in producing the protein myelin, which covers the nerve. This protective sheath breaks down if not enough vitamin B-12 is present.

Depression

In a busy Portland, Maine medical practice that combines conventional medicine and natural and preventive therapies, almost 75 percent of new patients have been prescribed antidepressants by prior health care providers. In the 1990's prescriptions for antidepressants increased 600%, and drugs such as Prozac, Paxil, Zoloft, Celexa, Lexapro, Wellbutrin, Effexor and Serafem are prescribed routinely for stress, headaches and minor depressions. Physicians under pressure from managed care systems find this to be a cost-effective solution with relatively little short-term risk. Without costly tests to determine causal factors, doctors have few or no answers for problems such as fibromyalgia, endometriosis, and rheumatoid arthritis, all of which have been linked to hormone imbalance, and a prescription for antidepressants satisfies the cost-conscious HMO as well as the discomforted patient. For example, the only definitive diagnosis for endometriosis is surgical; Fibromyalgia is diagnosed with MRI, although false diagnosis is frequent.[7] These expensive treatments and diagnostic tools can be foregone, in the short or long term, by masking symptoms with antidepressants.

According to the National Institutes of Health, one fourth of Americans suffer from depression, and over twelve billion dollars are spent for antidepressants annually. The more we understand about the gut-brain connection, the clearer it is that nutrition plays a major role in depression. A meta-analysis of studies in 2010 showed a strong correlation between depression and obesity, both of which have a root of systemic inflammation. Our fat tissues release inflammatory cytokines, which play a role in insulin resistance and cardiovascular disease. They can also cause inflammation in the brain. Insulin resistance causes a cascading effect—insulin resistance causes sympathetic nervous system overstimulation, which increases cortisol levels, which causes the body to lose magnesium. This can lead to migraine headaches and insomnia.

The intake of refined sugar has a similar effect, causing excess glucose, which degenerates brain function and causes an overproduction of cortisol. Increased cortisol has been linked to weight gain. There has been an increase in sugar intake from 2 pounds a year in 1940 to 150 pounds a year in many of today's teens who drink daily soft drinks.

Systemic inflammation can also be caused by food intolerance, especially wheat gluten, dairy and nuts. People with celiac disease report higher levels of depression. Lactose [dairy] intolerance has been linked to malabsorption of tryptophan. This leads to a serotonin deficiency, clinical depression, anxiety, and ADD/ADHD. A similar reaction can be caused by high fructose corn syrup.

Vitamin deficiency including Vitamin D and selenium can contribute to depression. The metabolism of refined sugar uses up the body's vitamins and minerals, especially the B vitamins, which are vital for maintaining mood.

---

7   Management of Fibromyalgia Syndrome—Reply. *Journal of the American Medical Association*, Vol. 293(7), February 16, 2005. "A neurosurgeon rating the overall MRI in a blinded fashion judged that 47% of the patients with fibromyalgia and 50% of pain-free controls would be surgical candidates."

Improving Brain Function by Optimizing Gut Health

Serotonin is a monoamine neurotransmitter and is biochemically derived from tryptophan, the amino acid inhibited by glyphosate, the main ingredient in Roundup. Serotonin is primarily found in the gastrointestinal (GI) tract, platelets, and in the central nervous system (CNS) of animals and humans. It is popularly thought to be a contributor to feelings of wellbeing and happiness. Approximately 90% of the human body's total serotonin is located in the gut where it is used to regulate intestinal movements. The remainder is synthesized in serotonergic neurons of the central nervous system, where it has various functions. These include the regulation of mood, appetite, and sleep.

Serotonin also has some cognitive functions, including memory and learning. Modulation of serotonin at synapses is thought to be a major action of several classes of pharmacological antidepressants. No less than 90 percent of serotonin uptake is from the gut. Neurochemicals produced by gut bacteria including lactobacilli and bifidobacteria are actively absorbed in the intestines and found in the blood.

The current pharmaceutical antidepressants function as serotonin uptake inhibitors (SSRI's). Studies in England have demonstrated that supplementing with tryptophan or its derivative, 5-HTP, is as effective as antidepressants with a fraction of the side effects. Researchers suggest that more women than men suffer from depression due to the fact that men synthesize serotonin at a rate 52 percent higher than women. Low serotonin in women is associated with depression and anxiety, and in men it is associated with aggression and alcoholism.

Serotonin deficiency is associated with hormone imbalance—low estrogen in women and low testosterone in men; lack of light, exercise, vitamins and minerals; and the presence of chronic stress. One can enhance the production of serotonin with Omega-3 supplements or by eating cold water wild caught fish.

Another amino acid affecting depression is tyrosine, which is made from phenylalanine. A Netherlands study showed that supplementing with tyrosine for military cadets resulted in better performance and memory. A Massachusetts study found folate deficiency to be associated with depression. Folate is necessary for the body to make the enzyme that methylates homocysteine. Elevated homocysteine and low folate levels are associated with severe depression. Genetic differences may affect a person's ability to methylate, which increases the need for folate supplements, as well as vitamins B12, B6, and zinc.[8]

---

8   Information on depression from Patrick Holford's research published in *Optimum Nutrition for the Mind*, published in UK.

A study funded by the Spanish government's medical research office of over 10,000 subjects documented that those eating a Mediterranean diet are half as likely to develop depression. The senior author of the study published in the *Archives of General Psychiatry* stated "both cardiovascular disease and depression share common mechanisms related to endothelium function and inflammation."

Beth Reardon, director of nutrition at Duke University suggested five foods to improve brain health: Egg yolks for vitamin B, nuts and seeds for magnesium, cold water fish for omega-3 fatty acids, quinoa, spelt and barley for complex carbohydrates, and green tea for the amino acid L-theanine.

What About Wheat?

What are the neurological effects of wheat? Dr. F. Curtis Dohan observed that during WWII when there was a shortage of wheat bread, there were fewer hospitalizations for schizophrenia. The number increased when the war was over. He observed that in New Guinea where schizophrenia was unknown, when wheat products were introduced, it increased 65-fold. (*Wheat Belly*, p. 46). While working with the Veterans Hospital in Philadelphia, Dr. Dohan found that symptoms of schizophrenia were much improved when wheat was removed from the diet for four weeks, and the symptoms worsened when wheat was reintroduced.

There is now an explosion of processed food products requiring just a few pennies worth of basic materials. Wheat flour, cornstarch, high fructose corn syrup, sucrose, and food coloring are now the main ingredients of foods in the interior of every grocery store. Kraft's processed foods generate $48.1 Billion in annual revenues, an increase of 1,800 percent since 1980, most of which comes from wheat and corn snacks (*Wheat Belly*, p. 60). Finally, wheat is an appetite stimulant. It makes you want both wheat containing and non-wheat-containing foods. For some people, wheat is a drug, and its drug-like neurological effects can be reversed with medications used to counter the effects of narcotics, and eliminating wheat creates unpleasant withdrawal symptoms (*Wheat Belly*, pp. 53-54).

Brain Function and Gluten

Between 10 and 22 percent of people with celiac symptoms also have nervous system involvement. Cerebellar ataxia is a progressive problem with coordination that affects balance, and eventually basic self-care activities. The average age of onset is 50. Only limited recovery is possible, because brain tissue regenerates poorly, even when gluten is eliminated. Wheat intolerance can also affect the peripheral nervous system, which is often accompanied by diabetes. It presents as lack of sensation in the limbs, diminished control over blood pressure and heart rate, and poor muscle control. Gluten sensitivity is also identified with seizures, migraine headaches and stroke symptoms, but the studies associating neurological symptoms with gluten sensitivity are small and inconclusive. Yet as more is understood about the connection of gut health to brain chemistry, it becomes essential to examine the effects of new wheat on brain function.

Dr. Davis concludes by saying eliminating wheat, "this Frankengrain that has infiltrated every aspect of American culture," is not enough. You must eat real food—not highly processed, herbicide treated, genetically modified, ready-to-eat, high-fructose corn syrup filled, just-add-water food products. Kellogg's reaped $6.5 billion in breakfast cereal sales in 2010, and it spends a small portion of its massive profits funding "research" by dietitians and nutrition scientists, whose studies produce cereal-positive results which in turn influence the sympathies of media giants to their large advertisers in the cereal business. Can you really believe the American Heart Association's endorsement of Honey Nut Cheerios and Cocoa Puffs? "Eliminate wheat abruptly and completely," advises Dr. Davis.

Dr. Perlmutter, who reviewed over 250 studies in writing his book, Grain Brain, states that Alzheimer's deaths increased 68 percent between 2000 and 2010, which he blames on a lifetime of unhealthy grain consumption. Considering that the first Alzheimer's drug did not appear on the market until 1990, the rapid rise of this terminal illness is yet another indicator that drastic changes in our food and lifestyle in this generation have brought disaster not yet fully understood or documented.

Chapter 5 Recommendations

- Avoid refined sugar for its connection to depression, insulin resistance and vitamin depletion
- Beware of food intolerances that cause systemic inflammation, especially wheat and dairy.
- Eat foods high in selenium such as grass fed meats, seafood, nuts, and seeds.
- Get natural antioxidants from organic fruits and vegetables
- Get enough vitamin D through daily sun exposure and supplements.
- Our brain and digestive systems are intricately connected, and in constant communication via the vagus nerve. If the brain is not healthy, neither is the gut, and vice versa. Our gut produces antioxidant enzymes that protect the brain from free radicals
- Avoid exposure to heavy metals, high fructose corn syrup, pesticides, chemical fertilizers and other toxins
- Limit vaccines
- Vitamin supplements including B vitamins, folate, D-3 and selenium
- Avoid nitrates from processed meats such as bacon, hot dogs, and lunch meats
- Seek nutritional alternatives to antidepressants
- Balance hormones

Chapter 6
Natural Aging

The natural and normal pace of aging for all systems of the body is actually very slow, but accelerated aging can occur as a result of a number of factors. Most anti-aging doctors agree that being healthy and aging naturally hinges on being well nourished and absorbing what we eat; but that can be very difficult these days. Suzanne Somers says; "a number of factors contribute to the deterioration of the body--nutritional deficiencies are right at the top of the list…the food we eat is responsible for taking us up or taking us down. It is truly that simple."

Good nutrition keeps minds clear, hearts healthy, bones strong, hormones balanced, and skin radiant! In short, nutrition keeps all body systems operating at peak performance. Nutrition builds and maintains us from the cellular level up, but cellular function can also break down due to challenges like malnutrition, stress, hormone imbalance, toxic burden, and food additives, all of which cause inflammation. This "burn" causes aging of body systems to accelerate beyond what is a natural and normal level. Inflammation increases toxic burden, adding oxidative stress, all of which can negatively impact metabolism at the cellular level.

We routinely hear that asthma, acne, allergies, arthritis, herpes, reflux esophagitis, irritable bowel syndrome and many more health challenges and diseases have nothing to do with diet, but this is simply not accurate. Medical schools largely train healthcare professionals to prescribe and monitor the risks and effectiveness of medications. They typically have little or no scientific training in nutrition much less as a viable treatment modality, and they lack clinical experience in applying nutritional and lifestyle interventions. Yes dear reader, they simply don't know. If you wonder if this is so, take a look at your healthcare provider. Many of them are overweight and on the same medications being prescribed for you. It is sobering to be in a doctor's examination room and realize that you may actually know more than your doctor or nurse about health and wellness.

The problem with drug therapies is twofold. First, the cause of the disease is often not removed and a patient's disease process continues unaddressed. Second, the drugs too often add side effects, which can contribute to the deterioration of the patient's health and increase the risk of long-term dangers. Or simply stated: The cure is worse than the disease.

My clinical experience shows me that better nutrition and time will routinely resolve disease states, even though doctors often tell you (if diet is mentioned at all) your disease has nothing to do with what you eat, or that dietary changes won't help. Furthermore, a simple scan of medical literature corroborates my assertion that dietary changes are life changing--and for the better. So here's to good eating and better absorption. Let's get started!

You have either read carefully to this point or jumped to this section to learn what you can do to avoid the dangers of the Standard American Diet and a sedentary lifestyle. Hundreds of people have seen the difference with just a few simple changes a few at a time to restore their broken health and escape chronic disease and premature aging. Linda Jeffrey is one of those people who was very reluctant to believe there was something wrong with her or that she should or even could do something to remedy her failing health position and rapid aging. Her success story should not be rare.

Dr. Deanna

Aging and Energy

Life at the Cellular Level

All of us once thought disease conditions were passed genetically from one generation to the next, but we are learning this is most often not the case. Today it is a simple fact: your diet probably lacks good nutritional value, because the foods are simply not nutrient rich, especially if you are shopping the grocery's inside aisles where the food industry offers an array of processed, reformulated, or the latest genetically modified "frankenfoods" or because you would rather eat what "tastes good." Perhaps you continue to eat the dishes your mother lovingly prepared, but if she suffered with or died of a chronic illness like diabetes, heart disease or cancer you may also be on your way to developing the same "family" disease issues.

If this is where you are health-wise, then this section of the handbook can help begin to redirect your future health destiny. Yes genetic make-up plays a role, but you are not a victim to your genetic predispositions. Your activity level to a lesser degree, and more importantly what you eat will either pull those genetic triggers, or you can learn to avoid pulling the triggers on those chronic disease states that "run in the family."

Most of America eats the Standard American Diet (SAD) consisting of processed foods in boxes, jars, cans or paper wrapped sandwiches passed from drive through windows. We routinely eat in the car, on the run, and have lost the art and joy of preparing, sitting and savoring a meal with others. If this describes you, then you can be sure your body isn't likely to get the raw materials it needs resulting in your body aging at an accelerated rate and a diagnosable disease is looming in your future. Sadly for so many, when the diagnosis eventually comes, most people will not relate the cause of the disease back to their own lifetime of poor diet and lifestyle choices.

If you are nutritionally challenged, evidenced by being overweight and often little or no energy, is it just a lack of willpower? According to Dr. David Kessler, former commissioner of the U.S. Food and Drug Administration, over-eating may be more insidious. Dr. Kessler says food manufacturers

> *Reverse Aging with Diet*
>
> *The 2009 Nobel Prize was awarded to three scientists who discovered that the caps at the end of our chromosomes—the telomeres—are protected and even lengthened by a plant-based diet, moderate exercise and stress reduction. Telomere length in test subjects following this regimen increased an average of 10 percent over five years vs. a control group whose telomeres decreased in length 3 percent. A shortening of the telomeres is associated with aging, chronic disease, and dementia.*

understand the chemistry of salt, fat and sugar, and that an addiction can be created for their food products by triggering a "bliss" point in the human brain, which mimics a powerful drug addiction. In other words, for millions of us, the real problem is that modern food is impossible to resist.

Kessler - who is also professor of pediatrics, epidemiology and biostatistics at the University of California – says it all comes down to the "bliss point," foods that actually change brain chemistry and instead of satisfying hunger, the salt-fat-sugar combination will stimulate that diner's brain to crave more. For many, slogans like -- "Betcha can't eat just one" -- are scientifically accurate. The food industry's manipulates this neurological response, designing foods to induce people to eat more than they should or even want is particularly troubling, when thinking about how these foods impact the health of children as childhood obesity rates rise. Obesity is understood to be a killer - which makes weight management a key to overall good health and disease prevention.

How important is nutrition to cancer prevention? Dr. Bernard Levin of Houston's MD Anderson visited Louisville, Kentucky in September 2004, and was quoted as saying two thirds of all cancers can be prevented through diet and lifestyle changes. When asked what the American public needed to learn to prevent cancer, Dr. Levin replied, "health literacy…understanding more about biology, having some grasp of what makes us tick and things we can do to make ourselves healthier." So let's learn about nutrition and the disease process and what we can do to make ourselves healthier.

Inflammation: Antioxidants vs. Free Radicals

Suzanne Somers reports, after hundreds of interviews with doctors, this is the bottom line: we are cell producing beings and this process must continue. Cell dysfunction— an assault or disruption of this process--eventually culminates in disease as the body deteriorates. Simple measures like changing from Omega 6 to Omega 3 oils can drastically improve cell function and reverse the aging process. There is no drug that can do that.

A growing number of researchers report that the inflammation-aging connection is the single greatest cause of aging and age-related diseases such as heart disease, diabetes, Alzheimer's disease, arthritis, certain forms of cancer, diminished mental and physical energy, the loss of muscle mass, and wrinkled, sagging skin.

What then is inflammation and oxidation? One is like a burn and the other like rust, but both create free radicals at the cellular level. There are three types of inflammation. Acute inflammation is the first response to tissue injury. You get a cut or a bruise and the body responds with wonderful resources to the area to start the healing process. Then there is inflammation from foreign antigens: Foods, microorganisms, toxins and parasites are in this group. The body again responds wonderfully with resources to fight antigens, which is good. The third type is chronic inflammation where disease and damage is ongoing, and either injury or antigens overwhelm body systems. Inflammation is the body's attempt to heal and fight invasion, but when there is too much damage or relentless toxic exposure, inflammation goes out of control.

Oxidation helps create energy in the body, but if it gets out of balance, oxidation causes damage. Free radicals form, circulate and create oxidative stress. Oxidation, like rust, speeds aging and damages cells and tissues. Because oxidation causes damage to cells and tissues, it will trigger inflammation. And when inflammation creates free radicals, it will trigger oxidative stress. The two go hand in hand.

"Oxidation is a very natural process that happens during normal cellular functions," researcher Jeffrey Blumberg, PhD, professor of nutrition at Tufts University in Boston, tells WebMD. Yet there is a downside. "While the body metabolizes oxygen very efficiently, 1% or 2% of cells will get damaged in the process and turn into free radicals," he says.

> ### What Are Antioxidants?
>
> *"A family of vitamins, minerals and other nutrients – compounds produced by the body that occur naturally in many foods. Antioxidants work together in the body to maintain our health and vigor well into the late decades of life. They do this by protecting us from damage caused by free radicals…Scientists now believe that free radicals are causal factors in nearly every known disease…In fact, free radicals are a major culprit in the aging process itself…By controlling free radicals, antioxidants can make the difference between life and death, as well as influence how fast and how well we age… There is overwhelming scientific evidence demonstrating that those who eat a diet rich in antioxidants and take antioxidant supplements will live longer, healthier lives…"* - Dr. Lester Packer, The Antioxidant Miracle

"Free radicals" is a term often used to describe damaged cells that can be problematic. They are "free" because they are missing a critical molecule, which sends them on a rampage to pair with another molecule. "These molecules will rob any molecule to quench that need," Blumberg says.

The Danger of Free Radicals: "Upstream" Medicine

When free radicals are on the attack, they don't just kill cells to acquire their missing molecule. "If free radicals simply killed a cell, it wouldn't be so bad… the body could just regenerate another one," he says. "The problem is free radicals often injure the cell, damaging the DNA, which creates the seed for disease." When a cell's DNA changes, the cell becomes mutated. It grows abnormally and reproduces abnormally -- and quickly.

As early as 1992 *TIME* magazine reported about life at the cellular level and in particular how the chronic disease process works. The "remedy" to fast paced aging is antioxidants – which are vitamins. Dr. Packer in his book, The Antioxidant Miracle, says, "A steady regimen of anti-oxidants both on the body and inside the body coupled with lifestyle changes that include an antioxidant rich diet and moderate exercise, is an excellent way to do our part to prevent and protect ourselves from accelerated aging," which again all begins at the cellular level.

Dr. Packer identifies the superhero antioxidants as Vitamin A, C, E, Alpha Lipoic Acid, and CoQ10. If you give the body enough Alpha Lipoic Acid, the body will make the glutathione it needs. Glutathione is important to detoxify our bodies at the cellular level. These antioxidant vitamins must all be present and work in concert to get the optimal anti-inflammatory and thus anti-aging effect.

To know your level of inflammation, there are blood tests to use as indicators, C-Reactive Protein, for example. Decelerating inflammation is possible, and diet is the key factor. Dr. Perricone advises to avoid problem foods that cause a rapid rise in blood sugar, which releases insulin into the blood stream. The biggest problem is sugar and foods that quickly convert to sugar in the body like simple carbohydrates (also processed foods made from grains and vegetables, juices, milk, and other foods many of us once considered good nutrition).

Accelerated aging includes a process of sugars attaching to collagen producing a stiff sugar-protein bond and accumulating throughout the body. As Dr. Perricone says, that "glue" is present in our veins, arteries, ligaments, bones, and even our brains. Simply stated sugars and simple carbs contribute heavily to accelerated aging in every body system including our skin.

Dr. Hyman also talks about inflammation as an "upstream" factor. Hyman is determined to find the root causes of disease, and treating conditions before they are diagnosed diseases. He says, if inflammation and immune imbalances are at the root of most of modern disease, how do we find the causes and get the body back in balance? First, we need to identify the triggers and causes of inflammation. Then we need to help reset the body's natural immune balance by providing the right conditions for it to thrive.

As a doctor, my job is to find those inflammatory factors unique to each person and to see how various lifestyle, environmental, or infectious factors spin the immune system out of control, leading to a host of chronic illnesses. Thankfully, the list of things that cause inflammation is relatively short:

(1) Poor diet--mostly sugar, refined flours, processed foods, and inflammatory fats such as trans and saturated fats; (2) Lack of exercise; (3) Stress; (4) Hidden or chronic infections with viruses, bacteria, yeasts, or parasites; (5) Hidden allergens from food or the environment; (6) Toxins such as mercury and pesticides; (7) Mold toxins and allergens.

> *Essential Oils are able to penetrate through skin due to their small molecules. They are absorbed into the bloodstream, into the lymphatic system; encourage growth of new cells delaying the process of aging by eliminating old cells more quickly. Different oils affect different hormones allowing weaker cells to leave the body and the remaining cells are strengthened, thus delaying aging by encouraging new cells and eliminating old. Circulation can also be improved, pain relieved, fluid retention reduced, and nerves calmed.*
>
> *Living Foods, p. 139*

By listening carefully to a person's story and performing a few specific tests, doctors like Hyman can discover the causes of inflammation for most people.

Fats: Good and Bad

Fats are misunderstood and while "fat-free" diets were a fad a decade or so ago, we now better understand how important good fats are to our health and to our sense of wellbeing. Not all fats are created equal and there is a difference between the two – good and bad. Bad fats are the "trans fats" and saturated fats.

Mayo Clinic says trans-fat is made by adding hydrogen to vegetable oil through a process called hydrogenation. Once we used butter fat, tallow, lard and bacon fat, but with refrigeration and other "advancements" we now use other hydrogenated vegetable fats like shortening and margarine. In manufactured foods hydrogenated fats help them stay fresh longer and have a longer shelf life. Scientists aren't sure exactly why, but the addition of hydrogen to oil increases your cholesterol more than do other types of fats. Commercial baked goods — such as crackers, cookies and cakes — and many fried foods, such as doughnuts and french fries — often contain trans fats – and shortening and margarine can be high in trans fat. Saturated fats are found in animal products like beef, pork, butter, and other full-fat dairy products.

Good fats are vital and cholesterol is critical to all functions of the body, especially hormones and our neurological system. Our brain is made up of about two thirds fat, and it can break fatty acids into ketones as a fuel source. Ketones feed the brain and prevent brain atrophy, and a primary source of ketone bodies are the medium chain triglycerides (MCT) found in coconut oil.

However, the primary fuel your brain runs on is glucose. When diabetes or the pancreas stops proper insulin production necessary to regulate blood sugar, then your brain literally starves, as it is deprived of the glucose-converted energy it needs to function normally.

In Alzheimer's disease, a brain atrophy disease, this process appears to begin one or more decades before the symptoms become apparent. The brain starts to atrophy, or starve, leading to impaired functioning and eventual loss of memory, speech, movement and personality. Diabetics or those with weakened ability to manage sugar have a 65 percent increased risk of also being diagnosed with Alzheimer's disease.

Omega 3, 6 and 9: The FATS

Most people simply don't get enough Omega 3s and yet this fat is vital to mental attitude and brain support, says Dr. Mark Hyman, author of *Ultraprevention* and the man who guided Bill Clinton to health via a vegan diet after his serious bout with heart diseases. Hyman calls Omega 3 "The king of good fats that come from wild foods. The problem is 99% of us are currently deficient in these healthy, essential fats."

When naturopathic doctor Alan Logan was asked to name the most helpful food factor for good attitude and disposition, he said, "If I had to pick only one dietary factor that could change your psychological condition, Omega-3s would be number one."He points to data showing that the average person's brain is starved for the omega-3s found in seafood, whole grains, grass-fed beef, flax seeds, walnut oils, and dark leafy greens like kale and spinach. As he says, "The brain is 60 percent fat and come retirement age or sooner, if you haven't deposited enough of the good kind of fat—Omega-3s—there is a greater risk of mental disease."

When it comes to weight loss, the Omega-3s offer many benefits. A study at the Charles University in Prague found that women on a low calorie diet lost significantly more weight and had greater reductions in their body mass indices (BMIs) and hip circumferences when they took supplemental Omega-3. But even if you are not on a low calorie diet, remember, Dr. Perricone says, that "it takes fat to burn fat—Omega-3s will do the trick."

Detoxing: Internal and External

This handbook deals extensively with hormone balance, but the other step necessary to health restoration and maintenance is detoxing. In a series of books, Suzanne Somers has interviewed anti-aging cutting-edge healthcare professionals across the country. The books are informative and easy-to-understand guides with lists of doctors across the U.S. who practice anti-aging medicine and nutritional healing. Suzanne says, after getting your hormones balanced, detoxing is the second of eight steps to "wellness." Many spa and alternative health practitioners also agree.

Dr. John Peterson, author of "Our Stolen Future" says; the chemical hot spot is not an oozing swamp of toxic effluent: it's our bathrooms, kitchens, living and bedrooms loaded with EDCs, Endocrine Disrupting Compounds, found in synthetic chemicals like phthalates which mimic estrogen in the body and have the ability to interfere with hormone systems. "Pollution isn't something coming out of a smokestack. It's in us. It's become part of the background chemistry of our bodies. And it's accumulating. And it's accumulating quickly."

Further says Peterson, sixty years ago, only a few synthetic chemicals had been invented. The explosion of modern chemistry began in the era of the military buildup during the 1930s-40s. Chemists invented plastics, pesticides, solvents, degreasers, insulators, and other materials for defense and to feed more people. Since WWII, more than 85,000 synthetic chemical compounds have been commercially developed and released into the environment. These toxic chemicals are suspected of contributing to cancers of the breast, prostate, brain and testicles, lowered sperm counts, early puberty, miscarriages, and other reproductive diseases as well as diabetes, ADD, asthma and autism. Bisphenol-A [BPA], a chemical used in plastics, is so common and is linked to lower sperm counts, early onset of puberty, insulin resistance and diabetes, prostate and testicular abnormalities, etc.

The body's largest external detoxifying organ is the skin, and the internal detoxifying organ is the liver. The liver filters out toxins and chemically converts them so they may be eliminated safely, but if your liver takes in more toxins than it can eliminate, it malfunctions causing a variety of symptoms.

- **External signs of a sluggish liver** are: coated tongue; bad breath; a flushed facial appearance; excessive facial blood vessels; acne; psoriasis; eczema; oily skin; rosacea; yellow conjunctiva (eyes); red swollen itchy eyes; dark circles under the eyes; brownish spots and blemishes (liver spots); rashes and itchy skin; inability to lose weight. Digestive issues are also a sign of an overburdened liver: Gall stones and gall bladder disease; intolerance to fatty foods; intolerance to alcohol; indigestion; reflux; nausea; abdominal bloating; constipation; irritable bowel syndrome; and hemorrhoids.

- **Neurological and emotional signs of toxicity** can include: Depression; mood changes; anger and irritability; poor concentration and "foggy brain;" and recurrent headaches with nausea.

- **Immune dysfunction** is also a sign of toxicity: Allergies; sinus; hay fever; asthma; dermatitis; hives; fibromyalgia; chronic fatigue; chemical and food sensitivities; auto-immune diseases; and recurrent infections.

If you are toxic and your liver is sluggish, it is important to be on a good balanced eating plan, water drinking regimen, exercise, rest, etc., along with nutritional supplemental support. A good plan to accomplish a complete internal and external cleanse is to drink water; eat a healthy-clean diet; drink a detox tea 2-3 times a day to support the liver and kidneys; daily dry brushing; and take a soaking bath each night during the cleanse period.

Finally, if you are not having a bowel movement within an hour or so after you eat, that could rightly be called constipation. Author James L. Wilson says waste that doesn't eliminate can seep back into the system. It's important to have enough fiber to move through the gastro-intestinal tract and keep regular...

> *Daily fiber in your diet improves bowel motion and re-establishes normal bowel function and strengthens adrenal function. As the body's responses become more efficient, your liver often begins to detoxify more rapidly. This means that more toxic constituents are contained in the bile that is secreted by your liver and emptied into your intestinal tract for elimination.*
>
> *Fiber prevents bile from becoming toxic in your large intestine by binding with it and moving it along the digestive tract. In this way, fiber helps eliminate fat-soluble toxins from your body. Without sufficient fiber present, these poisons may be released from the bile and reabsorbed through your intestines.*
>
>   – James L. Wilson, N.D., D.C., Ph.D., *Adrenal Fatigue*, Smart Publications, Petaluma, CA, 2007, p. 203.

As you gently purge the body's waste management systems of toxins and impurities, make sure to get adequate fiber, protein, vitamins, and minerals. Vitamin B5 and C, copper, zinc, magnesium, and manganese, these according to Dr. Perricone, are the principle nutrients needed to repair any type of tissue damage, from serious wounds to unwanted wrinkles. For seasonal detoxifying it could be helpful to spend a few days including a colon cleanse supplement along with the daily detox tea and adequate fiber.

Detoxing: Here are the steps

 To start your detox, pick a week you are home and not traveling. Limit your diet to fish, veggies, and plenty of water. As you detox it is important to get enough fiber to eliminate toxins. These suggestions help your liver maximize its detoxing function, and you can also help your skin, so both detoxing organs are working together. It's a good idea to use a dry brush every day (and particularly while detoxing) before showering or bathing. Using circular motions, come up the legs, arms and back moving the brush toward the heart. This brushing moves the lymph system. When detoxing, dry brushing exfoliates and aids in eliminating toxins through the skin. The skin is the largest detoxing organ of the body and it works best when exfoliated. While detoxing, consider calling a massage therapist for a massage.

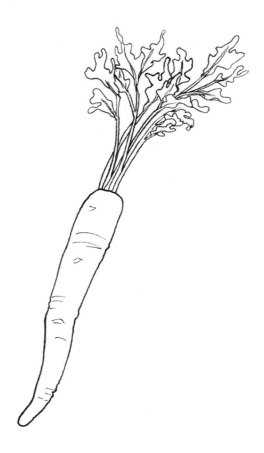

SKIN – Your Largest External Detoxifying Organ

The Brain-Skin Connection: Good for Your Skin, Good for the Brain

Dr. Perricone made an important link between skin and brain functions. He states:

> What is the exact connection between our brains and our skin? As a research scientist and a dermatologist, I have observed that if something has a positive effect on the central nervous system--whether it is a nutrient, herb, or any pharmacological agent--it seems also to have a positive effect on the skin. It all starts in the womb. The same layer of tissue from which the brain is derived is also the source of the skin. Consequently there is a strong connection between the two structures.

What goes on the skin can be absorbed through the skin via the two circulatory systems, the blood and the lymph, reaching every major organ of the body within seconds. Nicotine patches, for example, dispense nicotine via the skin. In the same way, putting antioxidants, vitamins, and good oils on the skin can have a positive impact upon brain health and function.

Back again to digestion and nutrition as a starting point: Dr. Perricone counsels, "You must provide your brain with the nutrients it needs to function at peak levels, to solve problems, to keep memory sharp, to generate creative ideas and to experience a state of well being." Your body needs a steady supply of high quality protein, because only protein satisfies hunger, and you must also have the right fats. What your body doesn't need is inflammatory foods like sugar and high-glycemic carbohydrates like wheat, pasta and potatoes.

Skin Types

Dr. Perricone categorizes skin types not as oily, normal or dry, but according to skin and hair color thus allowing him to develop skin regimens based on their potential for inflammation. Yes your skin can be inflamed and will age more rapidly due to adverse diet, lifestyle and environmental factors. Northern European skin – especially those of Irish and Nordic descent – lack melanin and experience much greater free radical damage when exposed to sun, than darker skin tones. Although sunlight exposure and dehydration can be a bigger problem for those prone to oxidative stress, they are less likely to scar or develop patches of discoloration and will heal beautifully with antioxidant support from cosmetic procedures.

African-American skin is not necessarily "thicker" or more resistant to drying, but the melanin rich skin, though often sensitive, is wonderfully protected from aging free radical damage. Vitamin C can reduce discoloration and scarring and normalize oily skin. Olive complexions are a tone between Northern European and African-American skin tones and tend to be more oily, which can make for a greater propensity to acne, enlarged pores, and blackheads. On the flip side olive skin is protected from the sun by melanin delaying the appearance of wrinkles, lines and sagging skin so prevalent in the lighter Northern European skin tones. Asian skin has more melanin than Northern European skin, but far less than African-American or Olive skin tones. Asian skin is resistant to sunlight and is at less risk for hyper-pigmentation seen in African American skin. Asian skin typically is neither chronically dry nor prone to acne, but their level of melanin content, Dr. Perricone says, leaves skin with little radiance. The underlying inflammation in Asian skin leads to water retention and edema that causes eye puffiness exaggerated by the Asian bone structure. A good skin brightener and increasing microcirculation of the skin will increase Asian skin radiance.

Finally exercise and fitness is a great boon to the immune system, mood, blood circulation and outwardly beautiful skin. Exercise, particularly resistance training, also produces Human Growth Hormone (HGH), an anabolic "youth" hormone which decreases levels of stress counteracting the destructive stress of the catabolic cortisol hormone. Bottom line--regular exercise can increase the secretion of HGH causing skin thickening and a radiant youthful appearance.

Sun & Skin

Vitamin D is vital to health maintenance. The sun is a source for Vitamin D, but there are variables affecting the body's ability to generate Vitamin D,which is a hormone instead of a vitamin. Dr. Richard Hobday explains in his book, *The Healing Sun*,that exposing a young white adult to a dose of sun long enough to cause a perceptible reddening of the skin, 24 hours after exposure, can produce as much as 10,000 IU of Vitamin D. In order to get the equivalent levels of Vitamin D, Asian and African skin need longer exposure times than white skin because of increased melanin content.

The elderly have a more difficult time converting sun exposure to Vitamin D. The skin of a 70 year old is 30 to 50 percent less able to produce Vitamin D than a 20 year old. There are some tips for sunbathing for health: Plan your exposure: don't cram sunbathing into 2-3 weeks of the year; frequent short exposures are better than prolonged exposures; don't bake in hot temperatures; the most important time of the year to sunbathe is spring and early summer; early morning sun seems particularly beneficial; to obtain the full spectrum of sunlight, don't cover with sunscreen or block; cover the thin sensitive skin of the face, head and neck; if you are sensitive to sun, begin with the feet, then legs, then abdomen, and chest; if you tan, tan gradually working up tolerance to sun; eat whole foods rather than refined foods; and no matter what, don't burn. If exposure to the sun is extended beyond that needed for Vitamin D production, then block or screen the sun with clothes or an SPF of no more than 30, anything beyond 30 can be chemically harmful.

Mineral Oil vs. Essential Oils

There is great benefit to essential oils, those pressed from living plants, while mineral oil is an inert (dead) substance, a byproduct of petroleum refining. Mineral oil is overwhelmingly used as the medium in U.S. personal care products because, bottom line, it is cheap. Mineral oil is occlusive, like a plastic wrapping on the skin. The skin is the largest detoxifying organ of the body and mineral oils, because of large molecules, make expressing toxins through the skin difficult. Mineral oil can block good skin function. Most U.S. companies use mineral oil as a medium in personal care products, while in many European countries it is banned for such use. Be sure to use personal care products without mineral oil as the medium.

Dr. John Lee said mineral oil is "estrogenic" and therefore not recommended for skin application. It just makes sense to use oils better suited for skincare. Essential oils are discussed in *Living Foods for Optimum Health*, written by directors of the Hippocrates Institute of West Palm Beach, Florida. Essential oils have the highest ORAC ratings of any substances in the world. The "ORAC" or Oxygen Radical Absorbency Capacity scale measures the antioxidant powers of foods and other substances.

According to Dr. Jordan Rubin, author of *The Makers Diet*, herbs and botanicals were humanity's first medical source. Herbs and spices are incredible sources of antioxidants with antimicrobial and anti-inflammatory properties…[that] still offer us medicines for inducing healing, preserving health and improving our quality of life. The Bible mentions at least 33 species of essential oils and makes over 1000 references to their use…essential oils were inhaled, applied topically, and taken internally. Some essential oils are antiviral and antibacterial, can re-program receptor sites in body cells and damaged DNA coding and are anti-carcinogenic.

According to Dr. Rubin who was stricken as a young man with Crohn's disease, essential oils have been highly prized since ancient times. Rubin reports: "four biblical essential oils greatly outperform the highest ranking fruits and vegetables in existence. For example, one ounce of clove oil has the antioxidant capacity of 450 pounds of carrots, or 120 quarts of blueberries or 48 gallons of beet juice." I am delighted to know that applying these wonderful oils and other antioxidants to my skin not only feeds my skin, but also aids cellular function which promotes health and well being overall, from head (the brain) to restoring and softening my toes and heels!

Essential oils work on the hypothalamus to actually change mood and attitude. Synthetically formulated perfumes alone or added to cleaning and personal care products may smell good, but that ends in the nose, because the scents don't work on the hypothalamus, and often cause allergic reactions.

_____

Chapter 6 Recommendations:

- Use a natural anti-aging skin care program free of petrochemicals, utilizing pure ingredients and essential oils
- Keep your body cleansed of toxins
- Avoid processed foods—the salt-fat-sugar complex
- Eat foods with a low glycemic index, clean and free of pesticides
- Use good oils in your diet: coconut, avocado, walnut, flax seed, and omega 3's
- Reduce inflammation with healthy antioxidants from organic vegetables and fruits
- Supplement with these antioxidants: Vitamins A, C and E, alpha lipoic acid, and CoQ10.
- Drink an average of 75 ounces of water per day

Chapter 7
Changing Diet and Lifestyle Patterns

Welcome to the practical application section of our handbook. This is where it all changes, because if you give the body what it needs and less of what it doesn't need, it will do the job it was designed to do. So where do I begin and what do I avoid? We invite you to use the handbook to answer questions, and to position you on the way to reclaiming your health and wellbeing.

What to Do in My Kitchen?
By Pam Leveritt

Pam Leveritt earned a BA from Ohio State University; is U.S. Army Veteran of Desert Storm; a graduate of Sullivan University; and serves on the Board of the Sensory Processing Disorder Support Group. Pam's goal is to help others become autonomous and confident in managing their kitchen spaces, from their refrigerators to their pantries with less stress and ultimately more success. Chef Pam provides guidance to transition to better nutrition. Let's here what Pam says about "restructuring" our kitchen and meal planning to answer the never-ending question of "What's for dinner?"

You may decide after reading all of the information in this book, or leaving the most recent doctor's visit just having been told that your diet must change due to allergies, diabetes, obesity, ADHD, etc. that you are very overwhelmed. Many families today find it hard to make drastic changes in their diets because they haven't been given the resources to be successful.

My daughter motivated me to transform my view of food, my kitchen, and my culinary training. At almost 7, she was diagnosed with SPD (Sensory Processing Disorder). We were shocked but I was strangely relieved because this would explain so many things like her being "a bull in the china shop" and running into things since age 3. Also labeled a "strong-willed" child, friends gave us James Dobson's, "The Strong-Willed

Child" to help us through this part of the parenting process. Did we just need to be better parents?

No one ever suggested that diet and food allergies could be contributing to our struggle. Commonplace were her complaints of itchy clothes, needing very tight squeezes and her intense cravings for sweets and carbohydrate packed foods. We reached out to the traditional treatment modalities for her symptoms, which included occupational therapy, vision therapy and the typical "sensory diet" which consisted of activities and toys that we could use outside of the therapy office to fulfill her need as a sensory-seeking child at home.

As she grew, it was evident there was more than a strong will. We were defining the symptoms, but not addressing the cause. There was something else. After a full evaluation, it was determined that she had a secondary diagnosis of ADHD and was highly sensitive to gluten, sugar and dyes to be specific. Then, as if we needed one more thing to worry about, the decision of "medication or no medication" was on the table. Kicking and screaming I agreed to meds because I finally realized that this was best at the time for our sweet girl.

I felt defeated when I finally conceded to medicating her. Why wouldn't I? Again, no one ever mentioned anything about nutrition as a healing method for SPD or ADHD. After struggling with the whole medication thing, it occurred to me that meds cannot be the only way to care for my child. Even as a trained chef, it did not readily occur to me that cleaning up our diet was vital to my child's health! Learning about the correlation between spectrum disorders and nutrition then became my focus. I joined a local SPD support group, which I am a co-facilitator of today, and just began to plug into everything that I could and read everything that I could get my hands on. It was exhausting but in the process I became friends with other parents who were going through the same thing. Every month we gathered together to talk about our atypical children and to learn from each other and to tell what their doctors and professionals were talking about. Not one word about nutrition.

The more I learned, the more I understood our eating habits HAD to change from the traditional SAD (Standard American Diet) of boxed macaroni and cheese and juice boxes to a cleaner and greener way of eating. I was greatly challenged, but over the last 5 years, we have managed to muddle through the world of Earth Fare and Whole Foods and have created a healthy and tasty diet that has completely changed our family from the inside and out.

A more plant-based whole food diet has been very positive for our daughter. Her medication has decreased to almost nothing, the intestinal imbalances in her gut have been healed and she has been able to think more clearly than ever. Today, if I *need a PowerPoint done, my now-brilliant 13-year-old daughter is the "go to" person at our house. Mind you, we have had our challenges large and small, but by taking control of our health and not following the SAD, we have overcome great obstacles by simply cleaning up our refrigerator and pantry and getting the junk out. By taking out the sugar, gluten, dairy and any prepackaged processed foods, we have significantly improved our health and wellbeing.*

We became a member of a local CSA (Community Supported Agriculture) where each week we support local organic growers and pick up a basket of seasonal vegetables. The CSA provides us the freshest and cleanest local food and our family sees the source of our food. Together we have learned to respect the food, something lost in our society today.

Today, more than ever it is necessary to learn as much as you can about the food you are consuming – read labels or stay away from "labels" and eat as fresh as possible. When I learn something new, I incorporate it into the life of my family. Most importantly in this process of food rediscovery, I am guiding our children on how to "eat to live" so they can prevent energy-sapping and life-shortening chronic disease in their lives. Prevention is the key to their success and yours. By changing your mindset, fleeing the "SAD," the physical, financial or emotional outcome will be far more rewarding than continuing on a path of less than optimal health. Thanks to my sweet daughter, my mission today is not to be a chef who cooks for others. My mission is to equip you with the tools and the guidance to choose good health for a long and vital life.

Here are my tips to assist anyone beginning a healthy eating change, whether by choice or necessity. I recommend a kitchen "assessment:" Look into your pantry, cabinets and refrigerator and purge food and equipment that clutter and halt the progress of achieving a healthier lifestyle for you and your family. This can all be stressful, but breaking it down into manageable tasks can achieve the desired result:

- **Assessment and Goal Setting:** Spend time with your family focusing on goals, wants, fears and stumbling blocks of each member to reach the nutritional goals of the family.

- **Pantry Check:** Remove food products that are prepackaged, contain harmful preservatives, dyes, colorings, sugars, starches and gluten, eliminating anything that is unnatural.

- **Organization:** De-clutter and simplify your kitchen and cabinet space keeping only what is necessary to achieve a functional kitchen. The more organized the space, the lower the stress of change.

- **Basic Cooking Techniques, Recipes and Ingredient Substitutions:** Modify family-favorite recipes to provide more nutritious versions of the old standbys; evaluate snacks and beverages; and employ cooking methods, such as roasting, steaming and baking, to replace less healthy methods.

- **Time Management:** Begin meal planning with a running grocery list. Shop and purchase local products. Adjust your schedule to allow meal planning which will bring the stress level down.

- **Shopping/Resources:** A change of diet requires a change of food purchasing patterns; purchasing from the best of markets; learning how to be thrifty, resourceful and creative in meal planning. Having a well-rounded stock of "go-to" recipes will make these nutritional changes much easier. There are websites and printed resources which will ease the frustration of managing your kitchen and prevent the possibility of being overwhelmed.

Thank you, Pam! Your story is helpful to many people today dealing with children and their sensory issues and neurological disorders. As you have read here, foods today are vastly different from those of even a generation ago. Resisting the question, "Now what do I do?" may be a stumbling block preventing a much needed dietary change. Asking for help may be difficult, but making these life-saving changes on your own may be too much for your busy lifestyle. Believe me, you will be so glad you made the changes. Choose a partner. It was the answer for Anna Joy and her mother Linda Jeffrey. With a lot of determination and patient guidance from Pam, here's what happened for them.

Two People Who Reclaimed Their Health
By Dr. Linda Jeffrey

I am an expert in grief, having learned as an unwilling student in a life shaken by sudden death, suicide, and devastating illness. I have been widowed three times, and have raised five children in the midst of earthquake-like life changes. So I understand firsthand how to live life appreciating the comfort value of food. I minister to grieving people and have written a book of encouragement entitled Comfort and Joy: How to Receive Healing beyond Grief and Loss. *Despite all of my extensive, formal education I was slow to understand the fact that grieving people too often use food to alleviate sorrows and loss. I did not realize that refined and processed foods are as addictive as cocaine and are a root cause of depression, only making losses more difficult to overcome.*

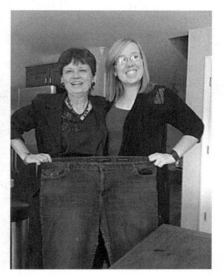

Two years ago, at the age of 57, I was struggling to maintain an active life as a writer, business owner, and mother of five. After a visit to the doctor, I was ominously advised to get my affairs in order, review my will and see a specialist because I was very sick. Arthritis had slowed my activity to the point that walking down the stairs was a major effort, and tying my shoes was impossible. I was a little concerned, but it had been so long since I had experienced health, I didn't know how sick I was. "It's menopause," my doctor said. You gain ten pounds a year, and your body and metabolism just slows down. It's to be expected." "We'll loosen you up with weekly visits," my chiropractor said. But the adjustments didn't help.

I thought we were healthy eaters, but our family bonding all centered on rich foods built from sugar and fat. Having been widowed three times, our family has been through many sudden changes, financial hardships, and the need to be close for each other. We got together regularly for family feasts, and were known as ones who knew how to entertain. Several months ago, my life changed radically. My daughter Anna Joy chose a health and wellness program that she dragged me into, along with her sisters and their families. Today we have collectively lost over 250 pounds, and we are at the phase of reflecting on what in the world happened to us, and why we didn't figure it out years ago!

Anna Joy, who was 17 and had fought a lifetime of obesity, asked me to change the way we eat. I agreed—but only for 30 days, and not one day longer! I loved my bread and ice cream after a hard day of work, and I thought I was signing on to misery—we had been on the diet merry-go-round many times. She simply asked me to give it 30 days. I consented, but only for 30 days!

A friend referred Chef Pam Leveritt to us. Pam came to our house and gently helped us clean out the refrigerator and pantry of refined sugar and bad oils, processed foods, and what I now know was just junk. We agreed to use a high quality vegan protein supplement for two meals a day to get our nutrition back on track and to give us time to learn to cook and eat another way. Without the shakes and homemade protein bars, I am not sure we could have made the transition from the way we knew to eat to a healthier program. We eliminated processed convenience foods containing sugar, dairy, wheat and bad oils from our kitchen. We learned how to cook our one meal a day, which was simply lean clean meat, with fresh and frozen vegetables and salads. Pam advised us to throw out the bottled salad dressings and showed us how to create salad dressings with healthy ingredients.

It turned into great fun to "partner" with Anna Joy as we learned how to make the changes to a healthful diet. With a fruit and protein shake in the morning, I was out the door in two minutes with a satisfying meal. The food tasted great, and I realized quickly that our grocery bill dropped dramatically! We were saving money! Around day seven, I realized I was walking up and down stairs without pain, and had much more energy. Something very dramatic was happening in my body. At the end of the second week with a seven-day cleanse of toxins, the weight loss accelerated for me. I had more stamina, clearer thinking, and NO arthritis pain. It then occurred to me how sick I had been, because for the first time in years, I finally understood what healthy feels like! My other daughters got on board, and when my son-in-law dropped seventy pounds, his dad and sister joined in, along with about thirty others for whom our extended family has shown the way.

Anna Joy, who has gone from a size 22 to an 8-10, is a bubbly positive health coach who now enjoys fashion and is charged with energy that had never been a part of her life. Genetics do not control or dictate a future of hypertension, heart disease, diabetes, and cancer. Our family has taken control of our future health, and it is amazing, easy, affordable, and permanent.

Finally for me this is a key piece of my ministering to those grieving and suffering loss. Yes spiritual resources are central to healing, but I now keenly understand the body also needs support and nourishment to sustain itself into the future and to really live again.

Transformation for Life - Age 19
By Anna Joy Jeffrey

Since I have struggled with weight my entire life and have been obese since age ten, I wasn't ready to jump in wholeheartedly in July of 2012, when a good friend came to me and said, "I want you to try this diet." She knew that throughout the years I had been a chronic dieter. You name the diet and I have tried it! I was so ashamed of how I looked and felt. I had reached a point of desperation. When she told me about a 30-day plan, I was finally willing to do just about anything to lose weight. I was tired of not participating in life because of my size.

The typical teenage activities were never a part of my life. I would go to theme parks and have to skip rides because the seats were not big enough for my body. I would sit in movie theaters and have to cross my arms not to bump the people next to me. I had to check weight limits for everything and I always felt like I was in the way. At my high school graduation I weighed two hundred and eighty-nine pounds. My prom dress was a size 22. Little did my friend know I was at a personal breaking point and had given up on ever being healthy and trim. I was resigned to be one of the many stories in the news media on obesity and diabetes in young people. I was petrified and sure I would die young because I was dangerously overweight. I had bought into the lie that the weight issues were genetic, and there was nothing I could do. After all, mother, when pregnant with me, had gestational diabetes, so I lived with the threat of also becoming diabetic.

At the age of eighteen, I was talking to my mother about weight loss surgery and stomach stapling, but my friend intervened and told me about an eating plan designed to help you bridge the gap from the addictive and mal-nutritious Standard American Diet [SAD] to a simple healthy diet. She showed me a vegan protein powder and told me to replace two meals a day with a vegan 20 mg protein shake, then focus on learning how to cook the one meal a day I was responsible for each day, for 30 days. One meal sounded completely manageable, so I was intrigued.

As we looked more into this product, I learned about the different types of protein and how they affect our bodies. I wanted to know why this plant-based vegan protein supplement was the best option. What we learned shocked us! When you go the grocery store to pick up a protein powder supplement, they usually come in two forms of protein: whey or soy. We learned that neither is good for your body.

Whey is a dairy derivative and the protein in dairy, casein, has been studied and linked in multiple research studies to tumor growth. In addition, according to a 2009 study reported in USA Today, about 60 percent of people can't digest milk protein, and I am definitely one of those people. Soy, on the other hand, is genetically modified and acts as a phytoestrogen in our bodies. This means that the soy we consume has an estrogenic effect once it passes your mouth. This can imbalance your hormones and affect every aspect of your health. A vegan protein supplement is the best choice because it is the easiest for your body to digest.

I knew for me to be successful I needed a partner and because I was living at home, who better than my mother? Mom wasn't thrilled about a new diet but she told me we could try the plan for thirty days, but if there was no difference by then, we were done! She was not excited about dieting…again!

The Plan:

Every day replace two meals a day with the vegan protein supplement and have one meal. I did a couple things with the protein supplement. I enjoyed protein shakes by blending together fruit and the protein powder and starting my day off with a smoothie. I also enjoyed making my own protein bars from the protein powder. The protein bars are great to pack and take to work and school with some fruit and nuts. When you consume your meal for the day, you eat clean by eliminating dairy, bad oils, sugar and gluten from your diet. If you eliminate these ingredients your body automatically knows how to process your food more efficiently and it will release the weight that you have been so desperate to lose.

My meal typically consists of four ounces of meat and lots of fruits and vegetables. When starting this plan, focus on counting your calories and staying under 1,250 calories in a day. This sounds crazy, I know, but I kept a food journal and documented every morsel that passed my lips. By writing down everything I ate, it kept me accountable and I was less tempted to eat junk foods. I found that my protein shakes only contained about two hundred calories and by the time I got to my one meal, I had six hundred to eight hundred calories to consume. I found that by the end of the day I struggled to hit one thousand calories! When you eliminate gluten, dairy, sugar and bad oil from your diet, you can eat more and consume less calories without being hungry. Only protein can satisfy hunger, and by drinking protein for your meals, you stay full and don't want to snack. On the occasions that you do feel the need to snack, you can snack on low sugar fruits or vegetables, or a bar made from pure protein powder.

About two weeks into this eating plan, I was introduced to Pam Leveritt, who helped guide me to success. Pam is a trained chef and her passion is teaching people how to eat and cook their food. She looked through our pantry and showed us the foods and condiments we needed to get out of the house because the chemicals in those foods were harming our bodies.

Simple carbohydrates that spike blood sugar wear the body out, weaken the immune system, and increase belly fat. We had to get them out of the house! We then went to the grocery and Pam taught us to shop the outside walls of the store and not to walk the isles. On the outside of the store you have fresh fruits, vegetables and meats and you are not tempted by walking past the baking section or the cereal section. Pam introduced us to several new spices that are also healing herbs, and add taste, not poison like MSG, the universal flavor enhancer in cheap junk food.

After Pam taught us a new way to access the grocery store, she showed us healthier cooking techniques. Pam helped me get set and ready to go! I watched Pam's website, and we began to try new recipes she posted, especially for homemade salad dressings. We limited our oils to walnut, coconut and avocado, and eliminated processed sugars all together. My mother and I started to mix together creations in the kitchen. It was exhilarating to concoct foods without the gluten, bad oil, sugar and dairy. We found that our palates changed and we could really taste and appreciate foods maybe for the first time. Within a very short time we started to feel the difference that clean eating makes.

 After a week of eating clean, I had lost seven pounds and I thought to myself, "Hmm, there is certainly something to this!" Over my first month I lost twenty-three pounds and at this point I had learned what I was eating affects much more than just obesity. I found that not only was I losing weight, I had more energy. I had not been a morning person before. I would roll out of bed, pour into my car half asleep and go to school. Any tests or quizzes that I took before ten o'clock were a disaster because I was not awake. When I changed my eating, I found that I could wake up in the morning and I had the energy needed to do better in my classes at school. Later I learned that my body was being worn down by the sugar I was consuming. Processed sugar is a depressant, and if I ever had "one of those days" I would reach for my "comfort food", sugar. The sugar would depress me in every way and in turn I would eat more sugar. The next day I would be a zombie walking out of bed because my body was so worn out from the nonfood that I was consuming.

In today's world sugar is marketed so heavily as a comfort food because it does create a chemical reaction in your brain and makes you feel better in the moment, but over time sugar becomes a low-grade addiction. Over my first six months on this new

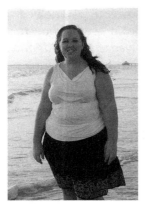

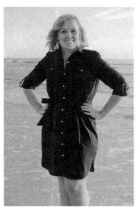

12 Month Transformation

eating plan, I lost over seventy-five pounds and it transformed my whole being. Now when I see friends I haven't seen for awhile, they ask what happened, because not only do they not recognize me physically, but I have changed. I have an excitement for life that was not there before I started on my reclamation of me.

I have learned more than anything that my body is a machine and it reacts to the fuel I offer. Now, I know if I eat foods harmful to my body, my body will react accordingly. Living this plan will never be over. I will continue to enjoy a protein shake for my breakfast and eat two meals clean of toxins, hormones, antibiotics and other foreign additives. Because I took 30 days to focus on learning how to cook one meal, I can now cook two clean meals with ease. If you would like to lose a few pounds, or would like to have more energy I challenge you to try this plan for 30 days. In reality, why stop yourself at thirty days? There is no limit to what you can do if you set your mind to it. I have completely reclaimed my life. I was on a path that, if I admitted it, was leading me straight to a life of disease, depression, misery and early death. I have chosen to be someone who will not only be a mother someday, but a grandmother who is healthy enough to dance at her grandkids' weddings. I recommend this plan to you to start your own health journey!

Exercise
with Tara Johnson

Diet comprises 85 percent of the health equation and exercise is 15 percent. Exercise is the smaller percentage, but it is still vital to your health position and cannot be left unaddressed in your new health program. Most people today struggle with good nutrition and adequate exercise due to a lack of knowledge, insufficient time and motivation. Why? Typically, the population doesn't get enough sleep leading to getting up "just in time" to go to work and/or get the kids to school. Then too often the domino effect occurs; we rely on caffeine instead of a healthy and nutrient rich breakfast; there is just no time for planning the rest of the day's nutrition and exercise; we grab a quick, fast and usually unhealthy lunch, followed by a afternoon snack, beverage, or both to get through the "mid-day slump;" then we have a large dinner because we have not eaten anything of substance all day. We end the day exhausted, and treat ourselves to the nightly snack as our reward for making it through another day. This leaves us full when we awake and the cycle repeats itself again...and again... and again. If only there was a plan, extra time and some motivation!

Let me introduce Tara Johnson. Tara earned her Bachelor of Arts degree in Sociology from Providence College in Canada where she was an All-Conference collegiate basketball player. As someone who has dealt with weight issues, Tara Johnson understands the commitment and dedication it takes to make changes in your life, then maintain them and stop the bouts of yo-yo dieting and exercise. She works with clients to set goals, develop a plan and modify behaviors to live a full and fit life. She is a certified personal trainer with the American College of Sports Medicine and owner of Get Fit for Life. If you would like to contact Tara 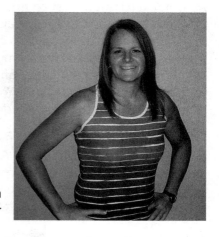 see the list of resources in the back of this handbook for contact information.

This section on exercise by Tara is included to help you develop a "Fat Burning Lifestyle" regimen for being healthy, strong and active.

Imagine that you were able to take a picture of the inside of your body. Right now, you could see the function of your heart, kidneys, lungs, liver, intestines, and colon. Would you look? Would you want to know if you were on the verge of developing high blood pressure, high cholesterol, diabetes and heart disease? What if you already have these diseases? Is medication your long-term plan?

As the doctors have already mentioned, these diseases are, in fact, caused by years of poor lifestyle habits. We neglect the one body we are given and when it begins to fail us, unfortunately, we don't get another.

Physical Fitness

The definition of physical fitness is the freedom from illness, infection, disease and shock and the ability to perform both vocational and recreational tasks without the risk of injury and undue fatigue. What would your life look like if you were the example, a model of physical fitness, according to this definition?

To make the journey manageable, I will break it down into 7 components of physical fitness: Aerobic exercise, Anaerobic exercise, Stretching, Low Body Fat, Realistic Nutrition, Proper Rest, and Stress Management.

Aerobic: Cardiovascular/Respiratory

Aerobic exercise is a must component of a healthy and balanced lifestyle and fitness program. It is necessary for a healthy heart and good respiratory care. Aerobic means in the presence of oxygen and is characterized by any activity that is performed at a low to moderate intensity for more than 60 seconds. This type of exercise allows oxygen to release energy through metabolism and can include running, jogging, walking, swimming and biking. You can use a treadmill, an elliptical, a stationary or recumbent bike or the great outdoors.

During an aerobic workout, the first 12-15 minutes you are burning sugar, then you enter into the fat burning stage. An optimal aerobic workout is 45 minutes and no longer than 60 minutes, unless you are an endurance athlete. For this type of exercise you will want to monitor your heart rate to ensure you are in the correct range and stay within this range for the duration of the workout.

To determine your range, use the simple calculation below:

- 220 - Age = Predicted Maximum Heart Rate (PMHR)
- Multiply your PMHR by 85 percent for your maximum base aerobic heart rate.
- Multiply your PMHR by 55 percent for your minimum base aerobic heart rate.

Use these two rates to determine your aerobic heart rate range. It is recommended to stay within this range once warm-up is complete and until cool-down begins.

There are several benefits of aerobic activity: increased cardiovascular function and a decrease in body fat. However, if aerobic activity is your sole type of exercise, keep in mind that there is potential for a decrease in muscle strength, muscle mass, power and speed. To minimize these effects, implement anaerobic exercise into your routine.

Anaerobic: Muscular/Skeletal Strength

Anaerobic by definition means without oxygen. Of course, this does not mean that you exercise without breathing. Put simply, anaerobic exercise is an activity that you complete at a high effort (90-110 percent of your PMHR) and have to stop to recover within 60 - 90 seconds. Your body is producing energy without utilizing oxygen. Anaerobic exercise is vital to build muscle, gain strength, and increase body tone. This type of exercise includes body weight resistance training such as push-ups, pull-ups and squats, free weights or weight machines and interval training such as running sprints.

During an anaerobic workout, your body uses two energy pathways. The first is high energy phosphates which are stored in very limited quantities within the muscle cell. This fuel source will sustain you for the first 5-10 seconds of the activity. Your body will then begin to use the second energy pathway, anaerobic glycolysis, where the body uses the breakdown of glucose for energy. This energy system produces lactic acid and leads to fatigue.

One of the best benefits of anaerobic activity is the after burn or excess post-exercise oxygen consumption (EPOC). EPOC refers to the oxygen consumption the body uses to return to its regular or pre-exercise condition. Remember, I have burned oxygen and high energy phosphates that need to be replenished and have produced lactic acid that the body must remove; not to mention resuming body temperature and blood circulation. The rate and duration of EPOC is dependent on intensity of activity, duration of exercise and continuous versus interval exercise. Studies have shown that the higher the intensity, the longer the duration and the more intervals all increase the rate of EPOC. Some research shows that EPOC after anaerobic activity can last between 12 and

Stress Management

High cortisol levels are associated with excess body fat and are raised by excessive stress. Stress is defined by Hans Sayle as any stimulus that places an adaptive demand on the systems of the mind and body. By this definition, stress is not inherently bad and can be something that is productive for us. However, our bodies begin to break down when the level of stress goes beyond our capabilities and limits. Fortunately, physical fitness increases your metabolic rate and burns off the harmful effects of stress, both emotionally and physiologically, while at the same time naturally contributing to hormone balance.

18 hours compared to 2 to 6 hours for aerobic activity. The longer the after burn, the greater the calories burned as you continue on with your day.

There are other benefits to anaerobic exercise: increased cardiovascular function, decreased body fat, increased muscle mass, improved strength, power and speed. One benefit of anaerobic exercise that is overlooked is an increase in aerobic capacity. When you utilize the anaerobic energy pathways, the aerobic pathways benefit also. Unfortunately, there is one catch associated of anaerobic exercise, it requires an aerobic foundation.

So, as I continue the balance theme, know that you must incorporate both aerobic and anaerobic exercise into your life. It is not an either or routine. The goal of any exercise prescription should be to optimize your performance in all aspects of physical activity.

Stretching: Joint Flexibility and Body Elasticity

Stretching may be the most important aspect of physical fitness and the most neglected. Flexibility is defined as the body's ability and freedom to move unrestricted through a joint's range of motion. Elasticity is defined as the body's ability to return to its original shape or condition before it was stretched. Most people don't build this component into their exercise regimen and fail to realize that stretching increases body strength and muscle tone.

There are different ways to stretch, with the most common being static stretch or static flexibility. This is a range of motion that can be achieved by holding a body stretch in a stationary position for a period of time. The primary purpose of this stretch is to relax a muscle and joint group. If you are trying to improve your flexibility, the best time to actively static stretch is at the end of the workout or when the muscle tissue is at a high thermal temperature. The best way to achieve the benefits of static stretching is to hold the stretch for a minimum of 20 to 30 seconds, but no longer than 60 seconds, as the benefits will not increase.

Prior to an exercise or stretching routine, a warm-up lasting at least 5 minutes should be implemented. This warm-up allows the muscle tissue's temperature and blood flow to increase. Including a warm-up pre-exercise or stretch will greatly reduce the risk of injury. The warm-up can include low intensity aerobic exercise such as walking or biking or a low intensity dynamic exercise such as skipping or jumping jacks.

If you are looking for a simple and effective exercise program, I recommend a 4-day split. This will require setting aside a minimum of 4 days per week for exercise. Here is how it breaks down:

- 4 days of anaerobic or strength training followed by aerobic or cardio training. It is important to complete your strength training before you perform any cardio, so you can use the energy stored in your muscles to lift the heaviest weight possible.

- The duration of each will be dependent on how much time you have available, but should include no more than 50 percent of your time performing cardio training.

- Remember to spend a minimum of 5 minutes warming up before starting a workout.

- You will have one rest day or an optional cardio training day in the middle of the 4-day split.

- You will have a second rest day or an optional leisure activity that needs to last a minimum of 30 minutes. This can include mowing the grass, playing basketball with your kids, going for a walk, etc.

- You will then set aside one day to completely rest and give your body time to rejuvenate.

The following layout is to be used as a guide.

	Sun	Mon	Tue	Wed	Thu	Fri	Sat
Anaer-obic	OFF	Strength - Upper body	Strength - Lower body	Rest	Strength - Upper body	Strength - Lower body	Rest
Aerobic	OFF	(Optional)	(Optional)	30-60 min (Optional)	(Optional)	(Optional)	30 min - Leisure activity (Optional)
Stretch-ing	OFF	5 min	5 min	5 min	5 min	5 min	5 min

Low Body Fat

As was stated in the introduction to this section, body fat and estrogen are intricately connected because fat cells produce estrogen. To achieve a proper hormone balance and great overall health, We must maintain our ideal weight and body fat percentage. Along with being a trigger for hormone imbalance, excess body fat is now recognized as a primary risk factor for coronary heart disease, cancer, diabetes, and autoimmune disorders by the American College of Sports Medicine.

To be clear, this section is titled "Low Body Fat", not "No Body Fat". Body fat serves several vital functions.

- Insulation - We need fat to keep us warm

- Cushion - We need fat as a layer of protection

- Fuel - We need fat to give us energy to move and exercise

- Transportation - We need fat to move vitamins and minerals throughout our body

With that said, how much fat is enough? The American Council on Exercise provides the following chart for reference.

Description	Women	Men
Essential fat	10–13%	2–5%
Athletes	14–20%	6–13%
Fitness	21–24%	14–17%
Average	25–31%	18–24%
Obese	32%+	25%+

One thing to consider when determining where you should be on this chart is body type or somatotype. There are 3 different somatotypes: Ectomorph, Endomorph and Mesomorph. Whether you are male or female, having an understanding of your body type will help clarify where you should fall in the range of body fat percentage.

- Ectomorph - characterized by smaller, lengthy bones and a struggle to add muscle mass

- Endomorph - characterized by a pear shape frame, larger bone structure and a higher total body mass

- Mesomorph - characterized by medium sized bones, athletic structure and a significant amount of lean muscle.

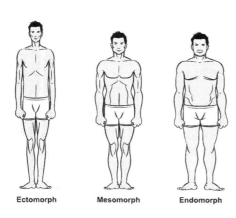

Ectomorph   Mesomorph   Endomorph

Knowing your body type can provide greater understanding of what your ideal body fat should be. For example, if you are a female Ectomorph, your body fat could be between 16-21 percent to be healthy compared to a female Endomorph who would still be considered healthy if her body fat fell between 21-25 percent.

It can be difficult and expensive to get an exact measurement of your body fat percentage. There are many methods available, but most are inaccurate and unreliable. The gold standard is underwater weighing where your weight is compared while immersed in water to your weight on dry land. However, this can be very costly and not easily accessible. Using skin-fold calipers and electrical impedance devices are highly variable and almost of no use because of operator error, liquid intake prior to measurement and the female's cycle.

One method for determining body fat is to use the Body Mass Index (BMI). This chart, which was invented between 1830 and 1850, uses your current height and weight to assess an individual's body weight from what is normal or desirable for a person of his or her height. The BMI does provide ranges from severely underweight to 3 levels of obesity, however everyone should remember that these are only statistical categories that should be viewed as a guide. You can find a copy of the Body Mass Index or a BMI calculator online.

If you need to lose weight, you must create a caloric deficit, meaning that you expend more energy (calories) than you are bringing in. One pound of body mass is equal to 3500 calories, so to lose 1 pound per week, you must create a caloric deficit of 500 calories per day. I highly recommend utilizing a food journal to record each calorie that is taken in. Most people have no idea how much food they are actually eating. If you are going to be successful at creating a deficit you must know what you are taking in. There are many smart phone applications and websites that make this task much easier. For most people, disciplining themselves to 1400-1600 calories per day will result in consistent and long-term weight loss. The diet needs at least 60 grams of protein per day, with healthy clean fruits, vegetables, good fats and a small amount of complex carbohydrates. For most people, eliminating sugar, wheat, and processed foods will accomplish the goal. Typically, you will want to lose 1-1.5 pounds per week. This will ensure that your body is adapting to long-term change and increases your odds of sticking with it.

Another vital key to health is hydration. You must be drinking half of your body weight in ounces of water every day. For example, if you currently weigh 150 pounds, you will need to drink 75 ounces of water per day. There is 70 percent water consistency in our bodies and most of us live in a constant state of dehydration. Water hydrates your body and provides the medium for proper digestion, nerve firing and body communication. Besides, fat is not soluble in water, so water will push fat through cell walls, into the liver and kidneys for the process of excretion. Water is a must for overall health!

Proper Rest

Our bodies need rest in order to function at a high level during the hours we are required to be awake. Allan Holson, director of the Laboratory of Neurophysiology at Harvard states, "Consistent, high quality sleep is where our bodies and our minds recover, restore and grow from all of the events and circumstances of our lives that occurred the day before." Your body is doing amazing things while you sleep and for overall health, we must allow time for proper rest.

In his book *The Seven Pillars of Health*, Dr. Don Colbert gives five reasons why sleep and rest are so important for physical fitness and wellness.

- Sleep regulates the release of important hormones, such as Human Growth Hormone, or HGH, which regulates muscle mass and helps control fat and leptin, which directly influences appetite and weight control.
- Sleep slows the aging process.
- Sleep boosts your autoimmune system by releasing white blood cells during sleep that destroy viruses and bacteria.
- Sleep improves brain function.
- Sleep reduces cortisol levels raised by excessive stress. High cortisol levels are associated with an excess of body fat.

So, with all those benefits happening while you rest, it is recommended that you get 7 to 9 hours of sleep per night.

The Importance of Post-Workout Nutrition: Recovery Secrets
By Lanty O'Connor

Refueling the muscles after a workout is essential for any athlete looking to maximize gains and prepare for the next workout. If your muscles are not receiving the correct macronutrients, in the correct amounts, at the correct time, you are losing out on better performance. My experience is that most people don't properly refuel after a workout. Usually one (if not more) of three things happens:

- *Nothing is consumed after a workout*
- *The wrong things are consumed after a workout*
- *The timing of the recovery is incorrect*

So here's what you need to know about post-workout nutrition:

First, let's briefly discuss some exercise physiology. Glycogen is a major fuel source during a workout. Glycogen is stored in the muscles and in the liver. The more highly trained an individual is, the more glycogen is stored in the muscles. After a work-out, the glycogen reserves are highly depleted. Additionally, protein breakdown is also high after a workout. In a 1980 article it was discovered that protein is used for fuel at a much higher rate than is generally assumed. This means that after a workout, the body is in a depleted, catabolic state.

So how do we deal with this state of depletion and catabolism? The answer is insulin. Insulin is the master recovery hormone. High-glycemic index carbohydrates will maximally stimulate insulin to begin the process of refueling the muscles.

The timing of what you consume after a workout is essential. We know that glycogen levels are low and protein breakdown is high after a workout. It has been demonstrated that there is a window of 30 minutes after exercise that is optimal for refueling. During that time period, the body is most able to recover. Ingestion of carbohydrates during the 30 minute window maximally increases insulin levels which promotes glycogen restoration. Additionally, increasing levels of insulin after exercise increases an optimal hormonal environment and can serve as a potent stimulator of protein synthesis.

The 30 Day Transition: What to Eat and Why

Good nutrition is vital to good health. Giving the body what it needs and then keeping away from foods that are difficult to digest or just plain not good for us, like corn syrup, sugar, and simple carbs, will work to stop accelerated aging and bring about a higher level of body efficiency and energy. In selecting the elements and the "how-to" for this important section, I sought the able guidance of Barbara Beaty, who has her Ph.D. in nutritional counseling.

Along with Dr. Beaty and others, I have worked to bring this simple eating plan to you to assist you in reforming your food selections and food quantities throughout each day for optimum health results.

Many people don't realize that fatigue, foggy thinking, poor sleep, excess weight (especially around the stomach, hips and thighs) and even aging skin indicate nutritional deficiencies that can be reversed. Adopting a healthier lifestyle for you and your family can be easy to talk about, but difficult to start without a plan. The *30 Days to Feeling Fit* plan is simple to follow and therefore, simple to complete. Let's get started:

Eat Clean

Fitness requires eating organic whole foods, free of gluten, preservatives, additives, pesticides, hormones, antibiotics, artificial colors and flavors, and all other toxins, because food is either fuel or poison. Simply put, anything that can't be used as energy in the body is a toxin. Organic fruits and vegetables contain up to 40 percent more antioxidants than those conventionally grown. This plan will help you learn how to fuel your body for optimal health by eating clean, close to nature and TOXIN FREE!

Increase Nutrient Intake

Due to the overabundance of pre-packaged and fast food, many people today are overweight yet malnourished. They carry toxic fat while their bodies are starving for real nutrition. This condition can be reversed by eating whole foods and supplementing with nutrients to fill in possible deficiencies created by mineral deficient farm soils.

Eliminate Allergenic and Addictive Foods

Many people experience symptoms of premature aging or poor health and have no idea that the solution may be as simple as removing possible food allergens. This plan includes removing possible allergenic foods like gluten, dairy, soy and processed sugars. If you cringe at the thought of removing a certain food, chances are you are allergic to it. Generally speaking, the food you crave is the food that is killing you.

- **Dairy** - Despite the widespread notion that milk is healthy, drinking pasteurized milk is frequently associated with a *worsening* of health. Sally Fallon of the Weston Price Foundation states, *"Pasteurization destroys enzymes, diminishes vitamin content, denatures fragile milk proteins, destroys vitamin B12 and vitamin B6, kills beneficial bacteria, promotes pathogens and is associated with allergies."* Only 30 percent of the calcium in a cup of milk gets absorbed. You would get twice as much calcium from a cup of broccoli. Many green leafy vegetables are loaded with calcium.

- **Soy** - Phytoestrogens in soy can mimic the effects of the female hormone estrogen. These phytoestrogens have been found to have adverse effects on various human tissues. Drinking two glasses of soy milk daily for one month has enough of the chemical to alter a woman's menstrual cycle.

- **Refined Sugar** - Refined sugar has been stripped of all nutrients and drains and leaches the body of precious vitamins and minerals. Sugar taken every day produces a continuously acidic condition which affects every organ in the body. Initially sugar is stored in the liver. A daily intake of refined sugar makes the liver expand like a balloon. When the liver is filled to its maximum capacity, the excess sugar is returned to the blood in the form of fatty acids. These are stored (and seen) in the most inactive areas: the belly, the buttocks, and the thighs. In contrast unrefined sugar like cane sugar contains minerals the body needs.

- **Gluten** - Gluten is a family of proteins found in grains. They are thick and gooey and make things stick together when baked, instead of falling apart. It is estimated that 50 percent of the population has difficulty breaking down gluten in their intestines.

When the immune system recognizes gluten in the gut as a "foreign protein," it attacks and damages the intestinal wall, which in turn causes the intestines to swell with water creating bloating and/or a "pot belly." Eventually, the intestinal wall thins to the point that it starts absorbing things that should have been blocked causing an array of problems including:

Allergies: The tips of the villi in the intestines produce the enzyme that digests the lactose in milk. Since they're the first to go, the very first symptom of gluten intolerance you see may be a "milk allergy" that manifests itself as a stuffy nose and post-nasal drip that occurs whenever you consume dairy products.

Immune Function: The constant load on the immune system as it fights off foreign proteins in the digestive tract impairs its ability to do its job elsewhere. Meanwhile, clogged sinuses and unhealthy intestinal walls create a perfect home for harmful bacteria to multiply.

Adrenal Function: The constant adrenal load created by chronic inflammation of the intestines eventually leads to adrenal insufficiency or even adrenal exhaustion. As the adrenals become impaired, many other symptoms manifest themselves, including allergies, slow weight gain and a loss of energy.

Balanced Blood Sugar

Our recommended health plan encourages eating low on the glycemic index for many reasons. The high, moderate and low "glycemic index" is a measure of how a given food affects blood-sugar levels, with each food being assigned a numbered rating. The lower the rating, the more gradual the infusion of sugars into the bloodstream and the more balanced the blood sugar.

High glycemic meals cause you to feel hungry soon after you eat. Eating low glycemic meals reduces hunger cravings. When blood sugar goes up in response to a high glycemic meal a process called "glycation" takes place, which promotes thinning of the skin and wrinkles. It's not just candy bars and cupcakes that elevate blood sugar. Pasta, bread, potatoes, white rice and other high glycemic fruits are also responsible.

Support Elimination Organs: Liver, Kidney, and Intestinal

As you repair fitness and health through good diet and nutrition, it would be incomplete if it did not support the body's five elimination pathways: the liver, kidneys, intestines and your largest detoxifying organ, your skin. It is nearly impossible to avoid the toxins we come in contact with on a daily basis. If toxins enter your body faster than they are removed, you will experience signs of toxicity. If, on the other hand, you give your body the support it needs to eliminate these toxins, it will perform optimally.

We wouldn't think about going a day without brushing our teeth, let alone years and years. Because we can't see our liver, kidneys, and intestines we forget the important role they play in detoxification. The liver has over 500 functions and the kidneys filter 200 quarts of blood per day. You can hold 5-25 pounds of waste in your large intestine (colon). All elimination organs need a "tune up" and proper maintenance.

A good detox tea assists the daily cleansing of the liver and kidneys by helping the body to filter and clear toxins. This in turn regulates cholesterol, balances blood sugar and promotes weight loss. Many are unaware that liver dysfunction is more closely related to obesity than any other single factor.   An overburdened liver is one of the reasons people plateau during weight loss.

Also helpful is a detox regimen to help cleanse and detoxify the system and support the liver, kidneys, and gastrointestinal (GI) tract. This assists with the gentle elimination of heavy metals and other environmental toxins.

Soaking 30 minutes in a bath of sea salts or mineral salts and essential oils literally draws toxins and heavy metals through the pores of the skin. Aches and pains will melt away and you'll find yourself sleeping better at night. For thousands of years people have enjoyed the healing benefits of sea water.

Your skin is your largest detoxifying organ. It is designed to both absorb nutrients and release toxins. Many people are very careful about what they put in their mouth but don't consider the toxins they are putting on their skin every day. It takes only 26 seconds for the toxic ingredients in skincare to find their way into every organ of your body.

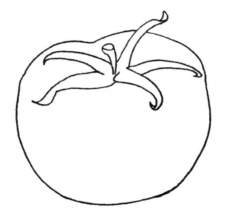

Clean Food Shopping Overview

Lean Proteins

When selecting meat, choose organic cage-free, hormone-free and free-range meats which are found in meat markets, health food stores or sometimes even at Costco. Only buy organic grass-fed beef and organic chicken. As for fish, purchase wild (never farmed) fresh or canned (in water).

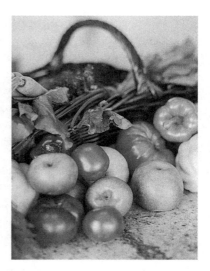

Free Range eggs come from hens that are allowed to grow and peck the ground. They are fed grain, seeds, and greens that contain a higher level of essential fatty acids than non-free range hens. Free range hens do not eat feed that has been treated with antibiotics and other chemicals.

A protein shake is a satisfying meal replacement, and can simplify the time and effort you are making to improve your health.

- **Why Is Protein So Important For My Regular Diet?**

  Protein is essential for growth and repair and makes up about 15% of the mass of the average person. Much of the human body is constructed from protein molecules, which play a crucial role in virtually all of the body's biological processes. Amino acids are the building blocks of protein. Some of these amino acids are produced naturally by the body; however nine amino acids are essential, meaning that the body does not make them and has to consume these amino acids from animal- or plant-food sources.

- **Which Protein Powder Should I Use?**

  The most common sources for protein powders are whey (a dairy or animal protein) and soy (a plant-based protein). Research on both soy and whey proteins reveal a number of related health concerns or side effects associated with their use:

  SOY – National Center for Complimentary and Alternative Medicine, a division of the National Institutes of Health, and the Harvard School of Public Health recommend individuals **limit** their soy intake to approximately 2-4 servings a week (16-32oz of soy milk or ½ cup-1 cup of tofu a week). Consuming large amounts of soy protein can provoke allergies, increase cancer risks, contribute to weight gain, lead to enlarged thyroid, and reduce the efficacy of some prescription medications. [8]

WHEY – Misconceptions about whey have lead bodybuilders to think they need large amounts of whey to succeed, when in fact, excess protein intake can result in abdominal pain, gas, bloating, and diarrhea. Additionally, whey protein is taken so easily that overindulgence is likely, leading to weight gain. As a milk derivative, whey is simply not an option for someone who suffers from milk allergies or lactose intolerance. The Mayo Clinic has warned that whey, like soy, can also have a negative effect on certain medications and other supplements. [9]

PEA PROTEIN - Most vegetable proteins are incomplete proteins and only offer a few essential amino acids, while animal proteins offer all essential amino acids and are considered complete proteins.   A PEA-based protein that provides a 100% amino acid score and supplies all essential amino acids from vegetable sources is an excellent source of protein. I recommend a pea protein that provides 20 grams of protein from different sources like pea, cranberry and rice proteins and is also therefore soy-, lactose- (whey), and gluten-free.

- **How Much Protein Is Enough?**

An average, a healthy adult needs 1 gram of protein per 2.2lbs of body weight per day (roughly half your body weight). For example, a 150 lb adult would need 70 grams per day divided between meals to meet daily basic nutritional levels and 20 grams of protein is nearly one meal's worth.

Weight Loss - My 30 Days detox and weight loss or reset program is designed primarily for weight loss by implementing nutritious meal replacements with Protein Shakes for 2 out of 3 meals each day for 30 days. Fiber is also important to add to increase your daily fiber intake and assist your liver in detoxing as your body reduces or resets if you are simply detoxing for 30 days.

Healthy Weight and Muscle Gain - For active men and women who regularly exercise, protein consumed within an hour after working out will provide amino acids for the building and repair of muscle tissue. To gain weight (especially muscle mass), simply continue eating normal meals and adding pea protein, ideally after the workout session for muscle recovery.

---

8   http://www.livestrong.com/article/249173-what-are-the-dangers-of-soy-protein/#ixzz1zlu6SfQy
9   http://www.livestrong.com/article/485624-problems-with-whey-protein/

Weight Management - If weight maintenance is your goal, shakes make a great breakfast or lunch on the go. Add fruits or veggies to make a smoothie.

Healthy Shakes For Children - Children can also benefit from pea protein, particularly when included in smoothies made with whole foods like spinach, kale, berries, avocado, or banana. For a 30 lb child, the recommended serving would be approximately 5 grams or a half scoop of Protein Powder.

- **NO ARTIFICIAL SWEETENERS – No GLUTEN**

I recommend a Pea Protein naturally sweetened with cane sugar and stevia, a natural herb with no side effects. However, many comparable products on the market save calories in their protein shakes by using artificial sweeteners, a popular solution for anyone counting calories to lose or maintain weight. But ironically, mounting evidence shows that artificial sweeteners, besides having many serious neurological side effects, may actually contribute to weight gain, increasing food cravings and instructing your body to store fat. [10] Look for nutrition and weight loss products are formulated without artificial colors, artificial flavors, artificial sweeteners, animal products, animal by-products, cholesterol, saturated fats and trans fats.

According to Dr. Mark Hyman, "Tricking your brain into thinking you are getting something sweet plays dirty tricks on your metabolism. Artificial sweeteners disrupt the normal hormonal and neurological signals that control hunger and satiety (feeling full). Alarmingly, Dr. Hyman references a study that found "rats offered the choice of cocaine or artificial sweeteners always picked the artificial sweetener, even if the rats were previously programmed to be cocaine addicts.

Healthy Fats

Use Extra Virgin Olive Oil (EVOO) in salad dressings and for low heat sautéing. Walnut oil can also be used in your homemade salad dressing recipe. Use Coconut Oil for high heat sautéing. Olive oil turns rancid (becomes toxic) under medium high heat, whereas Coconut Oil maintains its integrity when heated. Coconut oil is solid at room temperature. It is most often sold in jars alongside all the standard bottled oils. Avoid high-oleic safflower, corn and canola oils as they are highly processed. Corn, canola, and cottonseed oils are usually made from genetically modified plants that have been sprayed with Roundup. Enjoy small servings of avocado, coconut milk, olives, raw nuts and seeds.

---

10 http://articles.mercola.com/sites/articles/archive/2009/10/13/artificial-sweeteners-more-dangerous-than-you-ever-imagined.aspx

High Fiber Carbohydrates

- DRY PACKAGED - Legumes and grains such as brown rice are often packaged and sold in ethnic or health food sections of grocery stores. For example, cooked brown rice, diced veggies and EVOO makes a delicious grain salad.
- FROZEN - Look for cooked squash, artichoke hearts, lima beans and other vegetables.
- CANNED - Watch out for high sodium. Read labels and compare beans, artichoke hearts (in water), organic soups and organic broths.
- REFRIGERATED - hummus, salsa, rice tortillas, cooked lentils, grain salads and pesto.

We invite you to visit the website www.deannaosborn.com to print meal plan guides and shopping lists to carry to the store and keep in your kitchen. Plan ahead! It is key to your success!

Helpful Notes

Most supermarkets and grocery stores now have healthier food choices, organic brands and a designated aisle just for health food. Do not feel like you need a Health Food Store to find the food/ingredients you need to start your program. However, if you do have a local health food store, Whole Foods Market or Earth Fare nearby, it would be great to start your shopping there.

If you are going to a health food store to shop for the first time, make sure you have time to look around and plan on asking for help. Everyone that works in these stores is ready to help and is usually very knowledgeable.

When you make your shopping list for the first week, start with foods on the Clean Food Choices list that you already like. Ease into the program on food you are familiar with and enjoy eating. You WILL need to switch to cage free proteins, grass fed beef, organic high fiber carbohydrates, fruits and vegetables whenever possible. This way you are not ingesting toxins with the foods you eat.

Follow the meal plan when making your list. This makes it easier when going to the store the first time. A list keeps you on track, helps you remember everything you need and keeps you from feeling lost. This way if you need to ask for something, you know what it is and can ask for it by name.

Clean Food Choices

LEAN PROTEIN	Grass fed beef, organic poultry, eggs from free-range cage-free chickens
HEALTHY FATS	Raw nuts, seeds (no peanuts), macadamia nuts, freshly ground flaxseed, olive oil, olives, flaxseed oil, cod liver oil, avocado, coconut milk, almond milk, almond butter
HIGH FIBER CARBS	Squash (acorn, butternut, winter), artichokes, leeks, lima beans, okra, pumpkin, sweet potato or yam, turnips, legumes (black lentils, adzuki beans, cow peas, chick peas, french beans, kidney beans, lentils, mung beans, navy beans, pinto beans, split peas, white beans, yellow beans), brown rice, quinoa, hummus, millet
FRUIT GLYCEMIC INDEX	**Low GI:** Blackberries, blueberries, boysenberries, elderberries, raspberries, strawberries, sour green apple **Moderate GI:** Cherries, pears, apricots, melons, oranges, peaches, plums, grapefruit, pitted prunes, apples, avocados, kiwi, lemons, limes, nectarines, tangerines, passion fruit, persimmons, pomegranates **High GI:** (avoid during weight loss except after a workout) Bananas, pineapples, grapes, watermelon, mango, papaya
NON- STARCHY VEGETABLES	Arugula, asparagus, bamboo shoots, bean sprouts, beet greens, bell peppers, broad beans, broccoli, brussel sprouts, cabbage, cassava, carrots, cauliflower, celery, chayote fruit, chicory, chives, collard greens, cucumber, jicama (raw), jalapeño peppers, kale, kohlrabi, lettuce, mushrooms, mustard greens, onions, parsley, radishes, eggplant, endive, fennel, garlic, ginger root, green beans, hearts of palm, radicchio, snap beans, snow peas, shallots, spinach, spaghetti squash, summer squash, swiss chard, tomatoes, turnip greens, watercress

Food Focus: The Balanced Eating Circle

When planning your meals think of how you would place food on a plate.

Portion Size Guide

1/2	of the plate =	Non-Starchy Vegetables
1/4	of the plate =	Lean Protein (fist size) or Protein Shake
3/16	of the plate =	High Fiber Carbohydrates and Low Glycemic Fruits*
1/16	of the plate =	Healthy Fats

* Moderate and High Glycemic Fruits allowed after workouts or if not trying to lose additional weight

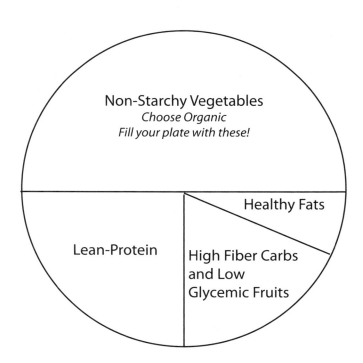

Simple Steps to Get Started

Day One

- Weigh yourself and record your waist measurements (at belly button and 2" below belly button)
- Go shopping and get prepared
- Get rid of all the temptations in your cabinets and fill your kitchen with healthy choices.
- Let your friends and family know what you are doing so they can support you for the 30 days!

Water is your best friend

- Drink at least six, 8 ounce glasses of water per day. If you get hungry, drink between meals.

Eat every 4 to 6 hours. Listen to your body.

- Do not go more than 6 hours without having a meal.
- No snacking except low-cal energy drink supplement, 1 teaspoon of almond butter or small handful of almonds. An exception is the "after workout recovery" shake to nourish your muscles. If having an after workout shake, your next meal is when you feel hungry.

Do not over eat when eating meals.

- Fill your plate with veggies. Add a fist size protein. Enjoy a healthy salad with homemade dressing.
- NO SECOND SERVINGS! Take your time eating.
- Chew your food.

Don't obsess over weight.

- Only weigh yourself 1 time per week - NOT EVERY DAY!

Have only healthy cleansing foods in your home/office.

Track your success.

- Write a food journal daily and keep a personal journal on how you feel each day.
- Keep track of your weight loss once a week.
- Try on clothes that were tight in the past.

A Sample Day

Wake-up

- Cup of detox tea

Breakfast

- Protein shake supplying 20 grams of soy-free, whey-free, complete amino acid profile protein, with water, coconut, rice or almond milk. Add fresh or frozen berries or veggies or 1 teaspoon of almond butter
- Add ½ to 1 scoop fiber
- Keep it simple if you are under time pressure. 20 grams of protein, a cup of frozen berries, and a cup of water in a single serving blender gets you out the door with a nutritious meal in less than a minute.
- Take nutritional supplements/multivitamins and minerals
- Pack protein bars to curb hunger and avoid temptations for junk.

Snack (optional)

- Energy drink containing B vitamins and antioxidants, free of sugar and artificial sweetener. If you need something more, have a small handful of raw nuts, seeds or a teaspoon of almond butter, or a homemade protein bar (see recipes section).

Lunch (4-6 hours after breakfast)

- A fist size of lean protein, non-starchy veggies, brown rice or other high fiber carbohydrates, a small amount of healthy fat or protein shake prepared as above.

Snack (see above)

Dinner – (4-6 hours after lunch)

- Fist size lean protein, non-starchy veggies, brown rice or other high fiber carb, small amount of healthy fat
- DO NOT EAT AFTER 7PM – HAVE A CUP OF DETOX TEA AFTER DINNER

What If?

I am hungry.

- Make sure you are getting a fist size of protein at every meal
- If your protein source is a shake, make sure you eat an abundance of non-starchy vegetables
- Make sure you are drinking enough water
- Drink your snacks – have some water with fiber, detox tea or vegetable broth

I am not losing weight.

- Some people will not lose any weight until the third week – Stay with it!
- Be sure you are not loading up calories in your shakes.
- Eat plenty of non-starchy vegetables

Why do I feel bloated after my shakes?

- Use a probiotic digestive aid in your shakes
- Reduce the amount of fiber you are supplementing

I am losing weight and don't want to.

- Add more calories and fat to your shakes
- Eat any fruit you desire
- Add a starchy carbohydrate to your meals (brown rice or quinoa).
- Put an extra scoop of protein in your shakes

I am constipated.

- Make sure you are drinking enough water throughout the day at least eight, 8 ounce glasses.
- Make sure you are getting enough vegetables
- Add ground flax seed or psyllium seed
- Try an herbal colon cleanse

The process of detoxifying can make you feel sluggish, physically and mentally. It's not unusual to feel worse before you feel better. The nutrition and digestive support you will receive from multivitamins, minerals, probiotics and enzymes will assist your body in eliminating toxins at a more rapid rate.

Shake & Protein Bar Recipes

Helpful Hints for Shakes

Magic Bullet or other single serving blenders work great to blend shakes.

- Freeze fresh fruit and veggies for future use.
- Add fresh spinach to shakes (won't taste it!)

The Basics of How to Make a Shake

- 2 scoops protein shake (Chocolate, Vanilla or both)
- ½ to 1 scoop fiber
- Ice (optional)
- ½ cup berries (optional) and/or
- ¼ cup spinach or squash (optional)

Mix with your choice of the following liquids:

- 1 cup water
- ½-1 cup coconut milk, rice milk or unsweetened almond milk
- Add 1 serving of fat:
- 1 tsp. almond, walnut, flax or coconut oil (no peanut butter)
- ¼ cup coconut milk or coconut water
- 1 TBS ground flax
- 1 TBS nuts
- ¼ avocado

Feel free to experiment with the consistency and ingredients in your shakes to your liking. More ice for thicker shakes.

Shake Recipes

Chocolate Almond Shake

- 2 scoops chocolate protein powder
- 1 scoop fiber (optional)
- 1 tablespoon almond butter
- water, ice

Chocolate Shake

- 2 scoops chocolate protein powder
- 1 scoop fiber
- water, ice

Chocolate Strawberry Shake

- 2 scoops chocolate protein powder
- 1 scoop fiber
- 1/2 cup strawberries
- water, ice

Vanilla Berry Shake

- 2 scoops vanilla protein powder
- 1 scoop fiber
- 1/2 cup frozen mixed berries
- water, ice

Chocolate Vanilla Shake

- 1 scoop chocolate protein powder
- 1 scoop vanilla protein powder
- 1 scoop fiber
- water, ice

Chocolate Vanilla Chai Shake

- 1 scoop chocolate protein powder
- 1 scoop vanilla protein powder
- 1 cup almond milk
- pumpkin pie spice

Pumpkin Pie Shake

- 2 scoops vanilla protein powder
- 1 scoop fiber (optional)
- 4 ozs pumpkin puree
- 1 cup almond milk
- 1tablespoon pecans
- pumpkin pie spice & stevia to taste

Savory Shake

- Heat veggies (broccoli, zucchini, cauliflower, squash, etc.)
- Puree veggies
- Add:
  - 2 scoops vanilla protein powder
  - 1 scoop fiber
  - 1 cup cooked grain, whole grain milk or broth.
- Blend

Benefits of Using Coconut Milk in Protein Shakes

- Helps the body maintain blood sugar levels
- Poor glucose tolerance may mean a deficiency of manganese in the body.
- Coconut milk is an excellent source of this essential mineral.
- Keeps blood vessels and skin elastic and flexible
- The mineral copper is critically important for many bodily functions.
- Together with vitamin C, it helps keep blood vessels and skin elastic and flexible.
- Assists in weight control
- Medium chain fatty acids in the coconut milk (MCTs) are used in the body for energy, as opposed to long chained fatty acids (LCTs), that are stored as fat. Medium chain fatty acids create "thermo genesis" in the body which increases metabolism and burns energy.

To find a store near you that carries fresh coconut milk in the refrigerator section go to: sodeliciousdairyfree.com/store-finder

Protein Bar Recipes

High Protein Low Carb Chocolate Protein Bars • 3 cups vegan Chocolate Protein Powder • 1 cup vegan Vanilla Protein Powder • 1 heaping Tbsp Almond Butter • 1 cup Coconut Milk	Mix all in food processor or by hand until dough ball forms. Place in a 9 x13 inch pan. Flatten out to all edges. Cut into 20 bars. Refrigerate. Each bar is 75 calories.
Mexican Chocolate Bars • 4 cups vegan Chocolate Protein Powder • ½ cup Pumpkin Seeds • 1Tbsp Cayenne Pepper • 1 Tbsp Almond Butter • 1 cup Coconut Milk	Mix in food processor until ball forms. Press into a 9x13 inch pan. Cut into 20 bars. The cayenne aids in better digestion and gives your lunch a kick.
Vanilla Protein Bars • 4 cups vegan Vanilla Protein Powder • 1 Cup Coconut Milk • 1 Tbsp Almond Butter • Cinnamon	Mix together in a food processor until ball forms. Press into a 9x13 inch pan. Cut into 20 bars. Sprinkle with cinnamon. To add a variety try adding different extracts to your mix. My favorites include almond extract, hazelnut extract, and orange extract.

Recommended 30-Day Nutrition Plan:
Total Body Care and Supplements

- **Progesterone – Transdermal:** Use a natural balancing cream made without mineral oil, free of colors and fragrance, in an air and light tight container that delivers 20 mg of USP bioidentical progesterone from a metered pump.

  It is recommended to use ¼ tsp. (1 pump) to ½ tsp. per day. One pump should be applied in the evening; two pumps should be divided, one in the morning, one in the evening. Apply cream to the soft tissues, such as the chest, inner arms, neck, face, palms of the hands, and soles of the feet. It is recommended to rotate applications to a different soft tissue with each usage.

- **Fiber** added to your daily food intake is important to soothe the colon and helps you to feel satisfied longer and supports balanced blood. Just twelve grams of fiber accounts for nearly half of the recommended daily amount and a flavorless blend of soluble fiber, which is largely undetectable, can be added to all foods and beverages, including protein shakes.

- **Herbal Detox Tea** is more than a beverage; some can be used as a remedy and for support of the liver and proper body function, as well as a daily "clean up." A tea with the following herbs can be very useful: Milk Thistle, (fruit), Peppermint, (leaf), Dandelion (root), Sweet Fennel (fruit), Elder (flower), Parsley (leaf), Walnut (leaf), UvaUrsi (leaf), Licorice (root).

- **A 7 - 14 Day Detox Body Cleanse:** Periodically, seasonally or monthly, cleansing the body of cellular waste and heavy metals while supporting the detoxifying organs and avenues – the liver, the skin, the lungs, and the colon is an important health maintenance measure as well as preparing the body for weight loss. Eat clean -- vegetables, fruit, lean meats along with a detox cleanse and no sugar, alcohol, or simple carbs.

- **Detox Soak:** Bath treatments have been used for centuries for assisting the skin, the largest external detoxing organ, in ridding the body of toxins.

- **Digestive Aid** with digestive enzymes, prebiotics and a probiotic to support the intestinal wall often damaged by allergenic foods. Probiotics scrub away yeast overgrowth in the lower GI and reestablish friendly bacteria.

- **Protein Shakes** that are vegan, made without dairy or soy, and free of gluten, no trans fats, artificial sweeteners, flavors or colors, are preferable. Drinking meals is easier on digestion and allows our body to have energy for detoxification and is useful as a quick and easy recovery shake after a workout.

- **Energy Drinks** can be used between meals to curb appetite without elevating blood sugar. An energy drink that promotes proper pH also aids in detoxification, but it's important the drink is free of sugar, artificial sweeteners and is low in calorie.

- **A Daily Multi-Vitamin and Multi-Mineral** with green tea, grape seed extract, cranberry extract, pomegranate extract, bioflavonoids, vitamins, minerals, herbs, antioxidants, digestive enzymes and probiotics is suggested. In addition to providing support for body systems during detoxing and for supplementing nutrition deficiencies from depleted soils, I like to see a high ORAC (Oxygen Free Radical Absorbent Capacity) score. An ORAC score of 10,000 is equivalent to eating 16 to 20 antioxidant packed fruits and vegetables.

- **Skincare:** Use only hair, body and skin care products free of mineral oil, harmful chemicals, and additives. Choose those with anti-inflammatory antioxidants rather than steroids as anti-inflammatories that may interfere with adrenal function.

Concluding Remarks From Dr. Deanna

After years as a family practitioner and seeing thousands of patients, I know good health requires work. It takes a clear decision by each of us to take charge of our own health position. I am delighted to offer you this handbook with just enough details so you can get in the driver's seat to maintain or regain health, maybe for the first time. Each one who has contributed to this book has a personal story that includes changing eating and lifestyle patterns for dramatic and permanent improvements in health. Following the simple steps in this handbook can make a huge difference in your life as well, in the health of your family, and has the potential to positively impact the world around you.

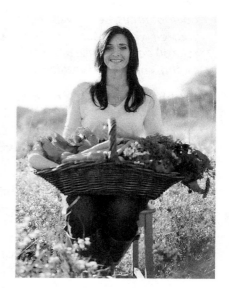

I have learned that traditional medicine doesn't always have all the answers, and sometimes the answers are just downright wrong. If I had followed the advice of traditional medicine, I would have had a hysterectomy five years ago and would probably be on multiple medications now. I chose a different path that led to health. I feel better now than I did even as a teenager! There are so many men and women out there that can learn from my experience and hopefully get back on track.

Why do you need to be in charge of your health? In today's busy medical practices, doctors simply don't have time to educate patients about health and/or diseases and their treatments. This handbook is intended to begin your health learning curve, so you can become an active participant, along with your doctor, in improving your health position. Health requires you to know your body better than anyone else. If you are certain something is just not right, then please, get "outside the traditional treatment box" and take time to read and research to get a better understanding, especially to learn what you can do.

The foundation of the guidance I offer is to first balance your hormones, which means clear, concise messages are being delivered to all your body systems; then cleaning up those body systems with a thorough, yet gentle, detoxing; add a good at-home exercise regimen, so you too can be fit without expensive gym fees. This coupled with proper nutrition and nutritional supplements provides a winning combination for health.

The material offered here is simple to understand, but so many of you may feel like you have so much to learn. So take your time. All who have started the journey to health have, at times, been overwhelmed. Start with one of the 4 sections and familiarize yourself with it. Master it, if you like, and then move to the next section. I believe it will take 30 days to make a transition from where you are to be solidly on the track to good health, energy and vitality.

Health and feeling fit is an exciting prospect and significant improvement is within reach. You can begin to see a difference right away. Initial success helps give us the heart needed to stay the course. Give me 30 days and I will show you how quickly changes can be made in your health.

The temptations are great and it is easier to let go and let others take responsibility for preventing disease, instead of maintaining our own health. Get outside the disease box that has us only seeking a remedy or treatment when a health issue arises and presses against us.

Finally, you can make a difference in the world around you. Become aware of the adverse effects that synthetic hormones are having on our environment. To ignore this issue, which is largely what our government has done, is ethically wrong and dangerous. Imagine our world 100 years into the future. Are men going to be exposed to such high quantities of estrogen that they are no longer able to reproduce, just as the male fish in the Potomac River have been feminized to the point that 30 percent of the male fish are able to produce eggs? If this comes about, we can expect changes for the human species as well.

I invite you to use this handbook to get ahead of disease and dysfunction and live life to its fullest. Together we can make a difference for ourselves, our children, and our children's children, by each one of us becoming healthier, developing water treatment systems that filter out pharmaceuticals, and by insisting that meat produced for human consumption does not contain growth hormones and antibiotics. It takes you to make a difference in your life and it takes only one person to make a huge difference in the larger world.

Dr. Deanna

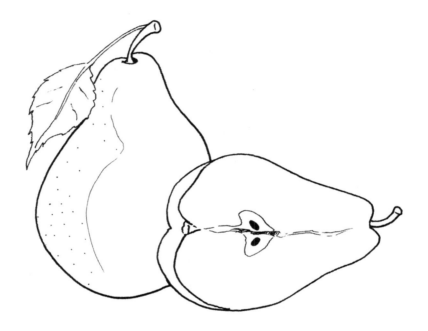

Helpful Websites:

www.arbonne.com
Vegan and organic products for the whole body.

www.annajoysjourney.wordpress.com
Anna Joy's story, blog and recipe website

www.breastreserachawarness.com
Informtion on breast health and thermography.

www.earthfare.com
Organic food supermarket offers in-store specials and recipes. Corporate headquarters in Asheville NC.

www.foodforlife.com

www.foodshouldtastegood.com

www.foxhollowfarms.com
Grass-fed Beef: Louisville, KY area

www.ushealthfoodstores.com
(find a store in your local area/state)

www.wholefoodmarkets.com
A wealth of information, do your research, make lists, get recipes, learn more or pre-shop before you enter the store.

www.zrtlabs.com
Saliva and blood spot testing.

Further Reading:

- Joseph Glenmullen, M.D. *The Antidepressant Solution: A Step-by-Step Guide to Safely Overcoming Antidepressant Withdrawal, Dependence, and "Addiction."* New York: Simon and Schuster, 2005.

- Dr. John Lee and David Zava, Ph.D. *What Your Doctor May Not Tell You About Breast Cancer.* New York: Time Warner, 2002.

- Dr. John Lee and Virginia Warner. *What Your Doctor May Not Tell You About Menopause.* New York: Warner Books, 2004.

- David Perlmutter, M.D. and Carol Colman. *The Better Brain Book.* New York: Riverhead Books, 2004.

- Barbara Seaman. *The Greatest Experiment Ever Performed on Women: Exploding the Estrogen Myth.* New York: Hyperion Books, 2003.

- Suzanne Somers. *The Sexy Years.* New York: Crown Publishers, 2004.

- Mark Hyman, M.D. and Mark Liponis, M.D. *Ultra-Prevention: The Six Week Plan That Will Make You Healthier For Life.* New York: Simon and Schuster, 2003.

- Dr. Don Colbert. *Toxic Relief.* Lake Mary, Florida: Siloam Press, 2001.

- Dr. Don Colbert. *The Seven Pillars of Health.* Lake Mary, Florida: Siloam Press, 2006.

- Michael R. Eades, M.D. and Mary Dan Eades, M.D. *Protein Power: The High-Protein/Low-Carbohydrate Way to Lose Weight, Feel Fit, and Boost Your Health – In Just Weeks!* New York: Bantam Books, 1999.

- Toni Weschler. *Taking Charge of Your Fertility: The Definitive Guide to Natural Birth Control, Pregnancy Achievement, and Reproductive Health.* New York: Harper Collins, 2002

- James Wilson.*Adrenal Fatigue –The 21st Century Stress Syndrome.* Petaluma, CA: Smart Publications, 2001.

- Dr. Linda Jeffrey, *Comfort & Joy: How to Receive Healing Beyond Grief and Loss.* Crestwood: Kentucky. First Principles Press, 2012.

Endnotes:

1 http://www.usc.edu/student-affairs/Health_Center/adolhealth/content/b3menses.
html#references

2 http://www.womentowomen.com/hormonalimbalance.aspx

3 http://66.241.252.6/images/femalehormon1.gif

4 Dr. John Lee, David Zava, Ph.D.: What Your Doctor May Not Tell You About Breast
  Cancer. New York, Time Warner, 2002, p. 53.)

5 Giovanni Brambilla and AntoniettaMartelli: Are some progestinsgenotoxic liver
  carcinogens? Mutation Research/Reviews in Mutation Research, Volume 512, Issues
  2-3, December 2002, Pages 155-163

6 A Bawde, WM Gregory, MA Chaudary et al,: Timing of surgery during menstrual cycle and
  survival of premenopausal women with operable breast cancer, Lancet 1991 (337):
  1261-1264. PE Mohr et al,: Serum progesterone levels at time of breast surgery and long
  term survival in node positive patients, Brit J. Cancer 1996 (73): 1552-1555.

7 Georges J. M. Maestroni (1993) The immunoneuroendocrine role of melatonin
  Journal of Pineal Research 14 (1) , 1–10 doi:10.1111/j.1600-079X.1993.tb00478.x

8   http://www.livestrong.com/article/249173-what-are-the-dangers-of-soy-
    protein/#ixzz1zlu6SfQy

9   http://www.livestrong.com/article/485624-problems-with-whey-protein/

10 http://articles.mercola.com/sites/articles/archive/2009/10/13/artificial-sweeteners-more-
   dangerous-than-you-ever-imagined.aspx

Bibliography

Bob Arnot, M.D. *The Breast Health Cookbook.* New York: Time Warner, 2001.

Bob Arnot, M.D. *The Prostate Cancer Protection Plan.* New York: Little, Brown & Co., 2000.

Paula Baillie-Hamilton, M.D. *Toxic Overload, A Doctor's Plan for Combating the Illnesses Caused by Chemicals in our Foods, our Homes, and our Medicine Cabinets.* New York: Avery Publishing, 2005.

Batmanghelidj, M.D. *Your Body's Many Cries for Water.* Vienna, VA: Global Health Solutions, 2004.

Sharon Batt. *Patient No More: The Politics of Breast Cancer.* Prince Edward Island, Canada: Gynergy Books, 1994.

D. Lindsey Berkson. *Hormone Deception.* Chicago: Contemporary Books, 2000.

Lee Bueno-Aquer. *Fast Your Way to Health.* New Kensington, PA: Whitaker House, 1991.

Brian Clement. *Living Foods for Optimal Health.* Roseville, CA: Prima Publishing, 1996.

Dr. Don Colbert. *Walking in Divine Health.* Lake Mary, FL: Siloam Press, 1998.

Dr. Don Colbert. *Toxic Relief, Restore Health and Energy through Fasting and Detoxification.* Lake Mary, FL: Siloam Press, 2001.

Dr. Don Colbert. *The Seven Pillars of Health.* Lake Mary, FL: Siloam Press, 2006.

Loren Cordain, Ph.D. *The Dietary Cure for Acne.* Fort Collins: Paleo Diet Enterprises, 2006.

Dementia and Testosterone Levels in Men. *Journal of the American Medical Association,* Vol. 293(5), February 2, 2005
W. John Diamond, M.D., W. Lee Cowden, M.D., Burton Goldberg. *An Alternative Medicine Definitive Guide to Cancer.* Tiburon, CA: Future Medicine Publishing, Inc., 1997.

Michael R. Eades, M.D. and Mary Dan Eades, M.D. *Protein Power: The High-Protein/Low-Carbohydrate Way to Lose Weight, Feel Fit, and Boost Your Health – In Just Weeks!* New York: Bantam Books, 1999.

Essential Oils Desk Reference. Essential Science Publishing, 2005.

Michael E. Gerber. *The E-Myth Revisited: Why Most Small Businesses Don't Work and What To Do About It.* New York: Harper Business, 1995.

Joseph Glenmullen, M.D. *The Antidepressant Solution: A Step-by-Step Guide to Safely Overcoming Antidepressant Withdrawal, Dependence, and "Addiction."* New York: Simon and Schuster, 2005.

Mireille Guiliano. *French Women Don't Get Fat.* New York: Alfred Knopf Publishing, 2005.

Drs. Scott C. Goodwin and Michael Broder. *What Your Doctor May Not Tell You About Fibroids.* New York: Time Warner Books, 2003.

Yashar Hirshaut, M.D. and Peter I. Pressman, M.D. *Breast Cancer, the Complete Guide.* New York: Bantam Books, 1993.

Richard Hobday. *The Healing Sun.* Scotland: Findhorn Press, 1999.

Mark Hyman, M.D. and Mark Liponis, M.D. *Ultra-Prevention: The Six Week Plan That Will Make You Healthier For Life.* New York: Simon and Schuster, 2003.

Mark Hyman, M.D. *The Ultra-Metabolism Cookbook.* New York: Scribner, 2007.

Jeffrey, Linda. *Comfort and Joy: How to Receive Healing Beyond Grief and Loss.* Crestwood: First Principles Press, 2012.

Alejandro Junger, M.D. *Clean Gut.* New York: Harper Collins, 2013.
Chris Kahlenborn, M.D. *Breast Cancer, Its Link to Abortion and the Birth Control Pill.* Dayton, OH: One More Soul Publishing, 2000.

David Kessler, M.D. *The End of Overeating. Taking Control of the Insatiable American Appetite.* New York: Rodale Press, 2009.

Michael Klaper, M.D. *A Diet For All Reasons* (video). Pauletter Eisen Nutritional Services, 1992.

Dr. Marysia Kratimenos. *Homeopathy Encyclopedia.* Boston: Octopus Publishing, 2003.

Dr. John Lee and David Zava, Ph.D. *What Your Doctor May Not Tell You About Breast Cancer.* New York: Time Warner, 2002.

Dr. John Lee. *What Your Doctor May Not Tell You About Pre-menopause.* New York: Warner Books, 2004.

John R. Lee, M.D., *Hormone Balance for Men: What Your Doctor May Not Tell You About Prostate Health and Natural Hormone Supplementation.* Dr. Lee cites the work of Dr. Calavieri reported in 1998 by the National Cancer Institute and available as NCI Monograph #27 from Oxford University Press.

Dr. John Lee and Virginia Warner. *What Your Doctor May Not Tell You About Menopause*. New York: Warner Books, 2004.

Janet Maccaro, Ph.D. *A Woman's Body Balanced by Nature*. Publisher's Recording, 1998.

Janet Maccaro, Ph.D. *90 Day Immune System Makeover*. Lake Mary, FL: Siloam Press, 2000.

Kathryn Marsden. *Good Gut Bugs, How the healing power of probiotics can transform your health*. London: Piatkus Publishing, 2010.

S. I. McMillen, M.D. *None of These Diseases*. Zenda, WI: Pyramid Publishing, 1963.

Dr. C. J. Mertz. *The World's Best Kept Health Secret Revealed*. Chiropractic Press, 2003.

Michael Murray, N.D. *The Complete Book of Juicing*. New York: Three Rivers Press, 1992.

Christiane Northrup, M.D. *The Wisdom of Menopause*. New York: Bantam Books, 2001.

Lester Packer, Ph. D. *The Antioxidant Miracle*. New York: John Wiley & Sons, 1999.

Leanne Payne. *The Broken Image, Restoring Personal Wholeness through Healing Prayer*. Wheaton, IL: Crossway Books, 1981.

David Perlmutter, *M.D. Grain Brain: The Surprising Truth About Wheat, Carbs and Sugar--Your Brain's Silent Killers*. New York: Little Brown and Co., 2013.

David Perlmutter, M.D. and Carol Colman. *The Better Brain Book*. New York: Riverhead Books, 2004.

Nicholas Perricone, M.D. *The Wrinkle Cure*. New York: Warner Books, 2001.

Nicholas Perricone, M.D. *The Perricone Prescription and Personal Journal*. New York: Warner Books, 2002.

Nicholas Perricone, M.D. *The Perricone Promise*. New York: Warner Books, 2004.

Michael Pollan. *Cooked, A Natural History of Transformation*. New York: Penguin Press, 2013.

Charles D. Provan. *The Bible and Birth Control*. Monongahela, PA: Zimmer Printing, 1989.

John Robbins. *A Diet for a New America*. Berkley: Publishers Group West, 1987.

Sherry A. Rogers, M.D. *Detoxify or Die*. Sarasota, FL: Sand Key Company, 2002.
Ron Rosedale, M.D. with Carol Coleman. *The Rosedale Diet*. New York: Harper Collins, 2004.

Ted Schettler, M.D. *In Harms Way: Toxic Threats to Child Development.* Boston Physicians for Social Responsibility, 2000. <http://psr.lgc.org/ihwrept/ihwcomplete.pdf>

Diana Scully. *Men Who Control Women's Health: The Mis-education of Obstetrician-Gynecologists.* Boston: Houghton Mifflin Co., 1980

Diana Schwarzbein, M.D.. *The Schwarzbein Principle: The Truth about Losing Weight, Being Healthy, and Feeling Younger.* Deerfield, FL: Health Communications, 1999.

Diana Schwarzbein, M.D. *The Schwarzbein Principle II.* Deerfield Beach, FL: Health Communications, 2002.

Barbara Seaman. *The Greatest Experiment Ever Performed on Women: Exploding the Estrogen Myth.* New York: Hyperion Books, 2003.

Suzanne Somers. *The Sexy Years.* New York: Crown Publishers, 2004.

Suzanne Somers. *Breakthrough, Eight Steps to Wellness.* New York: Crown Publishers, 2008.

Elizabeth Lee Vliet, M.D. *Screaming to be Heard: Hormonal Connections Women Suspect…And Doctors Ignore.* NY: M. Evans and Company, 1995.

Toni Weschler. *Taking Charge of Your Fertility: The Definitive Guide to Natural Birth Control, Pregnancy Achievement, and Reproductive Health.* New York: Harper Collins, 2002

James Wilson. *Adrenal Fatigue – The 21st Century Stress Syndrome.* Petaluma, CA: Smart Publications, 2001.

Index

E

F

G

H

I

More on the Authors

Dr. Deanna Osborn has completed the coursework leading to a Functional Medicine Fellowship. When as a young mother and physician she was struggling with serious medical issues, her field held no answers for restoring her health. Faced with her own health dilemma, Deanna discovered the importance of hormone balance, nutritional healing, and how simple lifestyle changes could restore her health. Dr. Deanna Osborn has proven that if you give the body what it needs or is lacking, it will heal itself. Today she practices part time in the area of Functional Medicine, specializing in bioidentical hormone balance, whole body detoxification, and the reversal of inflammation within the body.

Dr. Linda Jeffrey has discovered the secret of reversing debilitating chronic illness and accelerated aging using the principles in this Handbook. After a six-month experience during which she and her family collectively lost over 200 pounds, she began telling others about her restored health, weight loss, freedom from arthritis and other health issues. As a widow and grief counselor, she has written about the effects of grief on health and eating habits, and how restoring physical health is central to healing beyond grief. Dr. Jeffrey received her Doctor of Education from the University of Louisville in Curriculum and Instruction, and has earned a Master of Science degree and a Physician Assistant degree.

www.deannaosborn.com